This
KETO DIET JOURNAL
Belongs To:

....

Ketogenic Foods

MEATS

Beef
Sausage
Bacon
Lamb
Pork
Veal
Chicken/Turkey
Eggs

VEGGIES

Avocado
Asparagus
Argula
Broccoli
Cauliflower
Brussel Sprouts
Cabbage
Celery

VEGGIES

Cucumber
Chards
Bell Peppers
Green Beans
Collards
Mushrooms
Spinach
Olives

FRUITS

Blackberries
Cranberries
Blueberries
Lemon
Lime
Raspberries
Strawberries
Plantains (paleo)

DAIRY

Cheese (all kinds)
Sour Cream
Cream Cheese
Heavy Cream
Greek Yogurt
Almond Milk
Cashew Milk
Coconut Cream

CONDIMENTS

Balsamic Vinegar
Beef/Chicken Broth
Bonito Flakes
Tartar Sauce (keto)
Dijon Mustard
Mayo
Low Sugar Ketchup
Pickles

OILS & FATS

Avocado Oil
Butter
Coconut Butter
Duck Fat
Lard/Ghee
Nut Oils
Olive Oil
Pork Rinds

HERBS & SPICES

Garlic
Salt & Pepper
Oregano
Paprika
Cumin
Chili Pepper
Basil
Ginger

BAKING

Almond Flour
Almond Meal
Cashew Flour
Oat Fiber
Psyllium Husk
Whey Protein
Flax meal
Hazelnut Flour

FISH/SEAFOOD

Anchovy
Haddock / Cod
Halibut
Crab/Lobster
Mackerel
Salmon
Tuna
Red Snapper

DRINKS

Diet Soda (moderation)
Coffee
Tea
Gatorade Zero
Protein Shake
Club Soda
Broth
Coconut Water

MISC.

Canned Tuna
Pesto
Soy Sauce
Aioli
Béarnaise
Vinaigrette
Hot Sauce
Guacamole

NOTES:

Keto Grocery Inventory

DATE: _____

QTY	PRODUCE

QTY	MEAT & FISH

QTY	FROZEN FOODS

QTY	DAIRY

QTY	PANTRY

QTY	OTHER/MISC.

Macro Quick Reference

MACRO TRACKER

QTY	TYPE	PROTEIN	FAT	CARBS	CALS	NOTES

Keto Goals

1

USE THIS KETO JOURNAL AND DOCUMENT YOUR PROGRESS

COMPLETED ☐

2

CHOOSE 7 KETO FRIENDLY RECIPES TO TRY

COMPLETED ☐

3

CREATE A WEEKLY MEAL PLAN

COMPLETED ☐

4

WRITE DOWN EVERYTHING YOU EAT IN THIS PLANNER

COMPLETED ☐

5

PURCHASE A FOOD SCALE AND SPIRALIZER

COMPLETED ☐

6

TRY BULLET PROOF COFFEE

COMPLETED ☐

7

WEIGH YOURSELF ONCE A WEEK

COMPLETED ☐

8

GO ALCOHOL FREE FOR ONE WEEK

COMPLETED ☐

9

TRY A 12-HOUR INTERMITTENT FAST

COMPLETED ☐

10

CHECK AND LOG YOUR BODY MEASUREMENTS

COMPLETED ☐

11

LIST ALL THE REASONS WHY KETO WILL WORK FOR YOU

COMPLETED ☐

12

LEARN TO MAKE FAT BOMBS

COMPLETED ☐

13

MONITOR YOUR WATER INTAKE

COMPLETED ☐

14

INCREASE YOUR HEALTHY FAT INTAKE

COMPLETED ☐

15

TEST KETONE LEVELS USING STRIPS

COMPLETED ☐

KETO BEFORE & After

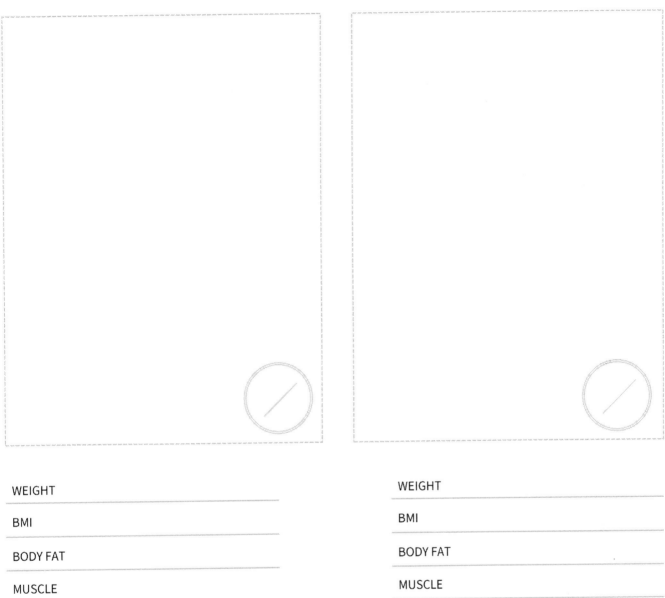

WEIGHT	WEIGHT
BMI	BMI
BODY FAT	BODY FAT
MUSCLE	MUSCLE
CHEST	CHEST
WAIST	WAIST
HIPS	HIPS
THIGHS	THIGHS
CALF	CALF
BICEP	BICEP
OTHER :	OTHER :
OTHER :	OTHER :

Weight and Measurements

Chest

Arm

Waist

Hips

Thigh

STARTING MEASUREMENTS:

| WEIGHT: |
| LEFT ARM: |
| RIGHT ARM: |
| CHEST: |
| WAIST: |
| HIPS: |
| LEFT THIGH: |
| RIGHT THIGH: |

My Journey

PERSONAL GOALS:

90 Days of Keto

Count down the next 90 days and track your progress!

STARTING WEIGHT:

DAY 90 WEIGHT:

1	2	3	4	5	6	7	8	9	10	LBS LOST:	INCHES LOST:
11	12	13	14	15	16	17	18	19	20	LBS LOST:	INCHES LOST:
21	22	23	24	25	26	27	28	29	30	LBS LOST:	INCHES LOST:
31	32	33	34	35	36	37	38	39	40	LBS LOST:	INCHES LOST:
41	42	43	44	45	46	47	48	49	50	LBS LOST:	INCHES LOST:
51	52	53	54	55	56	57	58	59	60	LBS LOST:	INCHES LOST:
61	62	63	64	65	66	67	68	69	70	LBS LOST:	INCHES LOST:
71	72	73	74	75	76	77	78	79	80	LBS LOST:	INCHES LOST:
81	82	83	84	85	86	87	88	89	90	LBS LOST:	INCHES LOST:

TOTAL WEIGHT LOST:

TOTAL INCHES LOST:

NOTES & REFLECTIONS:

21 DAY KETO *Challenge*

It takes just 21 days to create a healthy routine that will last a lifetime!
Let's stay in ketosis for 21 days!

START DATE	END DATE

1	2	3	4	5
6	7	8	9	10
11	12	13	14	15
16	17	18	19	20

21	NOTES

KETO GO TO *Meals*

BREAKFAST	LUNCH	DINNER	SNACKS
BREAKFAST	LUNCH	DINNER	SNACKS
BREAKFAST	LUNCH	DINNER	SNACKS
BREAKFAST	LUNCH	DINNER	SNACKS
BREAKFAST	LUNCH	DINNER	SNACKS
BREAKFAST	LUNCH	DINNER	SNACKS
BREAKFAST	LUNCH	DINNER	SNACKS

Favorite *Keto-Friendly Foods*

KETO FRIENDLY FOODS	NET CARBS	PROTEINS	FAT

FOODS TO EAT IN MODERATION	NET CARBS	PROTEINS	FAT

KETO Journal

MY KETO JOURNEY *Tracker*

SLEEP TRACKER:

DATE _____

 RISE: [   ] BEDTIME: [   ]   SLEEP (HRS): [   ]

NOTES FOR THE DAY

_____
_____
_____

EXERCISE / WORKOUT ROUTINE

TOP 6 PRIORITIES OF THE DAY

- ○
- ○
- ○
- ○
- ○
- ○

IN A STATE OF KETOSIS?

YES   NO   UNSURE

WATER INTAKE TRACKER

DAILY ENERGY LEVEL

HIGH	MEDIUM	LOW

BREAKFAST

FAT: CARBS: PROTEIN: CALORIES:

LUNCH

FAT: CARBS: PROTEIN: CALORIES:

DINNER

FAT: CARBS: PROTEIN: CALORIES:

SNACKS

FAT: CARBS: PROTEIN: CALORIES:

END OF THE DAY TOTAL OVERVIEW

CARBS	FAT	PROTEIN	CALORIES
[ ]	[ ]	[ ]	[ ]

DAILY FOOD *Journal*

FOOD TRACKER

MEAL/SNACK	NET CARBS	FAT	CAL	PROTEIN
DAILY GOAL:				
TOTAL:				

NOTES & MEAL IDEAS

MY KETO JOURNEY *Tracker*

SLEEP TRACKER:

DATE

 RISE:

ZzZ BEDTIME:

 SLEEP (HRS):

NOTES FOR THE DAY

IN A STATE OF KETOSIS?

YES   NO   UNSURE

WATER INTAKE TRACKER

EXERCISE / WORKOUT ROUTINE

DAILY ENERGY LEVEL		
HIGH	**MEDIUM**	**LOW**

BREAKFAST

FAT: CARBS: PROTEIN: CALORIES:

LUNCH

FAT: CARBS: PROTEIN: CALORIES:

DINNER

FAT: CARBS: PROTEIN: CALORIES:

SNACKS

FAT: CARBS: PROTEIN: CALORIES:

TOP 6 PRIORITIES OF THE DAY

END OF THE DAY TOTAL OVERVIEW

CARBS	FAT	PROTEIN	CALORIES
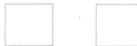

DAILY FOOD *Journal*

FOOD TRACKER

MEAL/SNACK	NET CARBS	FAT	CAL	PROTEIN
DAILY GOAL:				
TOTAL:				

NOTES & MEAL IDEAS

MY KETO JOURNEY *Tracker*

SLEEP TRACKER:

DATE _____

 RISE: | BEDTIME: | SLEEP (HRS):

NOTES FOR THE DAY

_____
_____
_____

IN A STATE OF KETOSIS?

YES   NO   UNSURE

WATER INTAKE TRACKER

EXERCISE / WORKOUT ROUTINE

DAILY ENERGY LEVEL		
HIGH	**MEDIUM**	**LOW**

BREAKFAST

FAT: CARBS: PROTEIN: CALORIES:

LUNCH

FAT: CARBS: PROTEIN: CALORIES:

DINNER

FAT: CARBS: PROTEIN: CALORIES:

SNACKS

FAT: CARBS: PROTEIN: CALORIES:

TOP 6 PRIORITIES OF THE DAY

- ●
- ●
- ●
- ●
- ●
- ●

END OF THE DAY TOTAL OVERVIEW

CARBS	FAT	PROTEIN	CALORIES
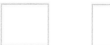			

DAILY FOOD *Journal*

MEAL/SNACK	NET CARBS	FAT	CAL	PROTEIN
DAILY GOAL:				
TOTAL:				

MY KETO JOURNEY *Tracker*

SLEEP TRACKER:

DATE _____

 RISE: _____   BEDTIME: _____   SLEEP (HRS): _____

NOTES FOR THE DAY

_____
_____
_____

EXERCISE / WORKOUT ROUTINE

TOP 6 PRIORITIES OF THE DAY

- ●
- ●
- ●
- ●
- ●
- ●

IN A STATE OF KETOSIS?

YES   NO   UNSURE

WATER INTAKE TRACKER

DAILY ENERGY LEVEL

HIGH	MEDIUM	LOW

BREAKFAST

FAT: CARBS: PROTEIN: CALORIES:

LUNCH

FAT: CARBS: PROTEIN: CALORIES:

DINNER

FAT: CARBS: PROTEIN: CALORIES:

SNACKS

FAT: CARBS: PROTEIN: CALORIES:

END OF THE DAY TOTAL OVERVIEW

CARBS	FAT	PROTEIN	CALORIES

DAILY FOOD *Journal*

FOOD TRACKER

MEAL/SNACK	NET CARBS	FAT	CAL	PROTEIN
DAILY GOAL:				
TOTAL:				

NOTES & MEAL IDEAS

MY KETO JOURNEY *Tracker*

SLEEP TRACKER:

DATE _____

| RISE: | BEDTIME: | SLEEP (HRS): |

NOTES FOR THE DAY

_____

_____

_____

EXERCISE / WORKOUT ROUTINE

TOP 6 PRIORITIES OF THE DAY

- ○ _____
- ○ _____
- ○ _____
- ○ _____
- ○ _____
- ○ _____

IN A STATE OF KETOSIS?

YES   NO   UNSURE

WATER INTAKE TRACKER

DAILY ENERGY LEVEL

| **HIGH** | **MEDIUM** | **LOW** |

BREAKFAST

FAT: CARBS: PROTEIN: CALORIES:

LUNCH

FAT: CARBS: PROTEIN: CALORIES:

DINNER

FAT: CARBS: PROTEIN: CALORIES:

SNACKS

FAT: CARBS: PROTEIN: CALORIES:

END OF THE DAY TOTAL OVERVIEW

CARBS	FAT	PROTEIN	CALORIES

DAILY FOOD *Journal*

FOOD TRACKER

MEAL/SNACK	NET CARBS	FAT	CAL	PROTEIN
DAILY GOAL:				
TOTAL:				

NOTES & MEAL IDEAS

MY KETO JOURNEY *Tracker*

SLEEP TRACKER:

DATE _____

 RISE: _____

BEDTIME: _____

 SLEEP (HRS): _____

NOTES FOR THE DAY

_____
_____
_____

EXERCISE / WORKOUT ROUTINE

TOP 6 PRIORITIES OF THE DAY

- _____   - _____
- _____   - _____
- _____   - _____

IN A STATE OF KETOSIS?

YES   NO   UNSURE

WATER INTAKE TRACKER

DAILY ENERGY LEVEL

HIGH	**MEDIUM**	**LOW**

BREAKFAST

FAT: CARBS: PROTEIN: CALORIES:

LUNCH

FAT: CARBS: PROTEIN: CALORIES:

DINNER

FAT: CARBS: PROTEIN: CALORIES:

SNACKS

FAT: CARBS: PROTEIN: CALORIES:

END OF THE DAY TOTAL OVERVIEW

CARBS	FAT	PROTEIN	CALORIES

DAILY FOOD *Journal*

FOOD TRACKER

MEAL/SNACK	NET CARBS	FAT	CAL	PROTEIN
DAILY GOAL:				
TOTAL:				

NOTES & MEAL IDEAS

MY KETO JOURNEY *Tracker*

SLEEP TRACKER:

DATE _____

 RISE: _____

 BEDTIME: _____

 SLEEP (HRS): _____

NOTES FOR THE DAY

_____

_____

_____

EXERCISE / WORKOUT ROUTINE

TOP 6 PRIORITIES OF THE DAY

- _____   - _____
- _____   - _____
- _____   - _____

IN A STATE OF KETOSIS?

YES   NO   UNSURE

WATER INTAKE TRACKER

DAILY ENERGY LEVEL

HIGH	**MEDIUM**	**LOW**

BREAKFAST

FAT: CARBS: PROTEIN: CALORIES:

LUNCH

FAT: CARBS: PROTEIN: CALORIES:

DINNER

FAT: CARBS: PROTEIN: CALORIES:

SNACKS

FAT: CARBS: PROTEIN: CALORIES:

END OF THE DAY TOTAL OVERVIEW

CARBS	FAT	PROTEIN	CALORIES

DAILY FOOD *Journal*

FOOD TRACKER

MEAL/SNACK	NET CARBS	FAT	CAL	PROTEIN
DAILY GOAL:				
TOTAL:				

NOTES & MEAL IDEAS

MY KETO JOURNEY *Tracker*

SLEEP TRACKER:

DATE _____

 RISE: _____   🌙 BEDTIME: _____   SLEEP (HRS): _____

NOTES FOR THE DAY

_____

_____

_____

EXERCISE / WORKOUT ROUTINE

TOP 6 PRIORITIES OF THE DAY

- ○ _____   ○ _____
- ○ _____   ○ _____
- ○ _____   ○ _____

IN A STATE OF KETOSIS?

YES   NO   UNSURE

WATER INTAKE TRACKER

💧 💧 💧 💧 💧 💧 💧 💧

DAILY ENERGY LEVEL		
HIGH	**MEDIUM**	**LOW**

BREAKFAST

FAT: CARBS: PROTEIN: CALORIES:

LUNCH

FAT: CARBS: PROTEIN: CALORIES:

DINNER

FAT: CARBS: PROTEIN: CALORIES:

SNACKS

FAT: CARBS: PROTEIN: CALORIES:

END OF THE DAY TOTAL OVERVIEW

CARBS   FAT   PROTEIN   CALORIES

DAILY FOOD *Journal*

FOOD TRACKER

MEAL/SNACK	NET CARBS	FAT	CAL	PROTEIN
DAILY GOAL:				
TOTAL:				

NOTES & MEAL IDEAS

MY KETO JOURNEY *Tracker*

SLEEP TRACKER:

DATE _____

 RISE:

BEDTIME:

 SLEEP (HRS):

NOTES FOR THE DAY

_____

_____

_____

EXERCISE / WORKOUT ROUTINE

IN A STATE OF KETOSIS?

YES   NO   UNSURE

WATER INTAKE TRACKER

DAILY ENERGY LEVEL		
HIGH	**MEDIUM**	**LOW**

BREAKFAST

FAT: CARBS: PROTEIN: CALORIES:

LUNCH

FAT: CARBS: PROTEIN: CALORIES:

DINNER

FAT: CARBS: PROTEIN: CALORIES:

SNACKS

FAT: CARBS: PROTEIN: CALORIES:

TOP 6 PRIORITIES OF THE DAY

END OF THE DAY TOTAL OVERVIEW

CARBS	FAT	PROTEIN	CALORIES

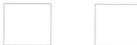

DAILY FOOD *Journal*

FOOD TRACKER

MEAL/SNACK	NET CARBS	FAT	CAL	PROTEIN
DAILY GOAL:				
TOTAL:				

NOTES & MEAL IDEAS

MY KETO JOURNEY *Tracker*

SLEEP TRACKER:

DATE _____

 RISE: _____

☾ᶻᶻᶻ BEDTIME: _____

 SLEEP (HRS): _____

NOTES FOR THE DAY

_____

_____

_____

IN A STATE OF KETOSIS?

YES   NO   UNSURE

WATER INTAKE TRACKER

💧 💧 💧 💧 💧 💧 💧 💧

EXERCISE / WORKOUT ROUTINE

DAILY ENERGY LEVEL		
HIGH	**MEDIUM**	**LOW**

BREAKFAST

FAT: CARBS: PROTEIN: CALORIES:

LUNCH

FAT: CARBS: PROTEIN: CALORIES:

DINNER

FAT: CARBS: PROTEIN: CALORIES:

SNACKS

FAT: CARBS: PROTEIN: CALORIES:

TOP 6 PRIORITIES OF THE DAY

- ● _____   ● _____
- ● _____   ● _____
- ● _____   ● _____

END OF THE DAY TOTAL OVERVIEW

CARBS	FAT	PROTEIN	CALORIES

DAILY FOOD *Journal*

FOOD TRACKER

MEAL/SNACK	NET CARBS	FAT	CAL	PROTEIN
DAILY GOAL:				
TOTAL:				

NOTES & MEAL IDEAS

MY KETO JOURNEY *Tracker*

SLEEP TRACKER:

DATE _____

 RISE: | BEDTIME: | SLEEP (HRS):

NOTES FOR THE DAY

_____

_____

_____

EXERCISE / WORKOUT ROUTINE

TOP 6 PRIORITIES OF THE DAY

○ _____ ○ _____
○ _____ ○ _____
○ _____ ○ _____

IN A STATE OF KETOSIS?

YES   NO   UNSURE

WATER INTAKE TRACKER

DAILY ENERGY LEVEL

HIGH	**MEDIUM**	**LOW**

BREAKFAST

FAT: CARBS: PROTEIN: CALORIES:

LUNCH

FAT: CARBS: PROTEIN: CALORIES:

DINNER

FAT: CARBS: PROTEIN: CALORIES:

SNACKS

FAT: CARBS: PROTEIN: CALORIES:

END OF THE DAY TOTAL OVERVIEW

CARBS	FAT	PROTEIN	CALORIES

DAILY FOOD *Journal*

FOOD TRACKER

MEAL/SNACK	NET CARBS	FAT	CAL	PROTEIN
DAILY GOAL:				
TOTAL:				

NOTES & MEAL IDEAS

MY KETO JOURNEY *Tracker*

SLEEP TRACKER:

DATE _____

 RISE: _____

🌙 BEDTIME: _____

 SLEEP (HRS): _____

NOTES FOR THE DAY

_____

_____

_____

EXERCISE / WORKOUT ROUTINE

TOP 6 PRIORITIES OF THE DAY

- _____ - _____
- _____ - _____
- _____ - _____

IN A STATE OF KETOSIS?

YES   NO   UNSURE

WATER INTAKE TRACKER

💧 💧 💧 💧 💧 💧 💧 💧

DAILY ENERGY LEVEL		
HIGH	**MEDIUM**	**LOW**

BREAKFAST

FAT: CARBS: PROTEIN: CALORIES:

LUNCH

FAT: CARBS: PROTEIN: CALORIES:

DINNER

FAT: CARBS: PROTEIN: CALORIES:

SNACKS

FAT: CARBS: PROTEIN: CALORIES:

END OF THE DAY TOTAL OVERVIEW

CARBS	FAT	PROTEIN	CALORIES

DAILY FOOD *Journal*

FOOD TRACKER

MEAL/SNACK	NET CARBS	FAT	CAL	PROTEIN
DAILY GOAL:				
TOTAL:				

NOTES & MEAL IDEAS

MY KETO JOURNEY *Tracker*

SLEEP TRACKER:

DATE _____

 RISE: | BEDTIME: | SLEEP (HRS):

NOTES FOR THE DAY

_____
_____
_____

IN A STATE OF KETOSIS?

YES   NO   UNSURE

WATER INTAKE TRACKER

EXERCISE / WORKOUT ROUTINE

DAILY ENERGY LEVEL		
HIGH	**MEDIUM**	**LOW**

BREAKFAST

FAT: CARBS: PROTEIN: CALORIES:

LUNCH

FAT: CARBS: PROTEIN: CALORIES:

DINNER

FAT: CARBS: PROTEIN: CALORIES:

SNACKS

FAT: CARBS: PROTEIN: CALORIES:

TOP 6 PRIORITIES OF THE DAY

- _____
- _____
- _____
- _____
- _____
- _____

END OF THE DAY TOTAL OVERVIEW

CARBS   FAT   PROTEIN   CALORIES

DAILY FOOD *Journal*

MEAL/SNACK	NET CARBS	FAT	CAL	PROTEIN
DAILY GOAL:				
TOTAL:				

MY KETO JOURNEY *Tracker*

SLEEP TRACKER:

DATE _____

 RISE: _____ 🌙 BEDTIME: _____ 💤 SLEEP (HRS): _____

NOTES FOR THE DAY

_____
_____
_____

IN A STATE OF KETOSIS?

YES   NO   UNSURE

WATER INTAKE TRACKER

💧   💧   💧   💧   💧   💧   💧   💧

EXERCISE / WORKOUT ROUTINE

DAILY ENERGY LEVEL		
HIGH	**MEDIUM**	**LOW**

BREAKFAST

FAT: CARBS: PROTEIN: CALORIES:

LUNCH

FAT: CARBS: PROTEIN: CALORIES:

DINNER

FAT: CARBS: PROTEIN: CALORIES:

SNACKS

FAT: CARBS: PROTEIN: CALORIES:

TOP 6 PRIORITIES OF THE DAY

END OF THE DAY TOTAL OVERVIEW

CARBS	FAT	PROTEIN	CALORIES

DAILY FOOD *Journal*

FOOD TRACKER

MEAL/SNACK	NET CARBS	FAT	CAL	PROTEIN
DAILY GOAL:				
TOTAL:				

NOTES & MEAL IDEAS

MY KETO JOURNEY *Tracker*

SLEEP TRACKER:

DATE _____

 RISE:

 BEDTIME:

 SLEEP (HRS):

NOTES FOR THE DAY

_____

_____

_____

EXERCISE / WORKOUT ROUTINE

TOP 6 PRIORITIES OF THE DAY

- ● _____   ● _____
- ● _____   ● _____
- ● _____   ● _____

IN A STATE OF KETOSIS?

YES   NO   UNSURE

WATER INTAKE TRACKER

DAILY ENERGY LEVEL

HIGH	**MEDIUM**	**LOW**

BREAKFAST

FAT: CARBS: PROTEIN: CALORIES:

LUNCH

FAT: CARBS: PROTEIN: CALORIES:

DINNER

FAT: CARBS: PROTEIN: CALORIES:

SNACKS

FAT: CARBS: PROTEIN: CALORIES:

END OF THE DAY TOTAL OVERVIEW

CARBS	FAT	PROTEIN	CALORIES

DAILY FOOD *Journal*

FOOD TRACKER

MEAL/SNACK	NET CARBS	FAT	CAL	PROTEIN
DAILY GOAL:				
TOTAL:				

NOTES & MEAL IDEAS

MY KETO JOURNEY *Tracker*

SLEEP TRACKER:

| RISE: | | BEDTIME: | | SLEEP (HRS): |

DATE _____

NOTES FOR THE DAY

_____

_____

_____

IN A STATE OF KETOSIS?

YES   NO   UNSURE

WATER INTAKE TRACKER

EXERCISE / WORKOUT ROUTINE

DAILY ENERGY LEVEL

| HIGH | MEDIUM | LOW |

BREAKFAST

FAT: CARBS: PROTEIN: CALORIES:

LUNCH

FAT: CARBS: PROTEIN: CALORIES:

DINNER

FAT: CARBS: PROTEIN: CALORIES:

SNACKS

FAT: CARBS: PROTEIN: CALORIES:

TOP 6 PRIORITIES OF THE DAY

- ○ _____   ○ _____
- ○ _____   ○ _____
- ○ _____   ○ _____

END OF THE DAY TOTAL OVERVIEW

CARBS	FAT	PROTEIN	CALORIES

DAILY FOOD *Journal*

FOOD TRACKER

MEAL/SNACK	NET CARBS	FAT	CAL	PROTEIN
DAILY GOAL:				
TOTAL:				

NOTES & MEAL IDEAS

MY KETO JOURNEY *Tracker*

SLEEP TRACKER:

DATE _____

| RISE: | BEDTIME: | SLEEP (HRS): |

NOTES FOR THE DAY

_____

_____

_____

EXERCISE / WORKOUT ROUTINE

TOP 6 PRIORITIES OF THE DAY

- ○
- ○
- ○
- ○
- ○
- ○

IN A STATE OF KETOSIS?

YES   NO   UNSURE

WATER INTAKE TRACKER

DAILY ENERGY LEVEL		
HIGH	**MEDIUM**	**LOW**

BREAKFAST

FAT: CARBS: PROTEIN: CALORIES:

LUNCH

FAT: CARBS: PROTEIN: CALORIES:

DINNER

FAT: CARBS: PROTEIN: CALORIES:

SNACKS

FAT: CARBS: PROTEIN: CALORIES:

END OF THE DAY TOTAL OVERVIEW

CARBS	FAT	PROTEIN	CALORIES

DAILY FOOD *Journal*

FOOD TRACKER

MEAL/SNACK	NET CARBS	FAT	CAL	PROTEIN
DAILY GOAL:				
TOTAL:				

NOTES & MEAL IDEAS

MY KETO JOURNEY *Tracker*

SLEEP TRACKER:

| RISE: | BEDTIME: | SLEEP (HRS): |

DATE _____

NOTES FOR THE DAY

_____
_____
_____

EXERCISE / WORKOUT ROUTINE

IN A STATE OF KETOSIS?

YES   NO   UNSURE

WATER INTAKE TRACKER

DAILY ENERGY LEVEL		
HIGH	**MEDIUM**	**LOW**

BREAKFAST

FAT: CARBS: PROTEIN: CALORIES:

LUNCH

FAT: CARBS: PROTEIN: CALORIES:

DINNER

FAT: CARBS: PROTEIN: CALORIES:

SNACKS

FAT: CARBS: PROTEIN: CALORIES:

TOP 6 PRIORITIES OF THE DAY

END OF THE DAY TOTAL OVERVIEW

CARBS	FAT	PROTEIN	CALORIES

DAILY FOOD *Journal*

FOOD TRACKER

MEAL/SNACK	NET CARBS	FAT	CAL	PROTEIN
DAILY GOAL:				
TOTAL:				

NOTES & MEAL IDEAS

MY KETO JOURNEY *Tracker*

SLEEP TRACKER:

DATE _____

 RISE: _____

BEDTIME: _____

 SLEEP (HRS): _____

NOTES FOR THE DAY

_____

_____

_____

EXERCISE / WORKOUT ROUTINE

IN A STATE OF KETOSIS?

YES   NO   UNSURE

WATER INTAKE TRACKER

DAILY ENERGY LEVEL		
HIGH	**MEDIUM**	**LOW**

BREAKFAST

FAT: CARBS: PROTEIN: CALORIES:

LUNCH

FAT: CARBS: PROTEIN: CALORIES:

DINNER

FAT: CARBS: PROTEIN: CALORIES:

SNACKS

FAT: CARBS: PROTEIN: CALORIES:

TOP 6 PRIORITIES OF THE DAY

○ _____   ○ _____

○ _____   ○ _____

○ _____   ○ _____

END OF THE DAY TOTAL OVERVIEW

CARBS	FAT	PROTEIN	CALORIES

DAILY FOOD *Journal*

FOOD TRACKER

MEAL/SNACK	NET CARBS	FAT	CAL	PROTEIN
DAILY GOAL:				
TOTAL:				

NOTES & MEAL IDEAS

MY KETO JOURNEY *Tracker*

SLEEP TRACKER:

 RISE:

BEDTIME:

 SLEEP (HRS):

DATE _____

NOTES FOR THE DAY

_____

_____

_____

EXERCISE / WORKOUT ROUTINE

TOP 6 PRIORITIES OF THE DAY

- • _____
- • _____
- • _____

- • _____
- • _____
- • _____

IN A STATE OF KETOSIS?

YES   NO   UNSURE

WATER INTAKE TRACKER

DAILY ENERGY LEVEL

HIGH	MEDIUM	LOW

BREAKFAST

FAT: CARBS: PROTEIN: CALORIES:

LUNCH

FAT: CARBS: PROTEIN: CALORIES:

DINNER

FAT: CARBS: PROTEIN: CALORIES:

SNACKS

FAT: CARBS: PROTEIN: CALORIES:

END OF THE DAY TOTAL OVERVIEW

CARBS	FAT	PROTEIN	CALORIES

DAILY FOOD *Journal*

FOOD TRACKER

MEAL/SNACK	NET CARBS	FAT	CAL	PROTEIN
DAILY GOAL:				
TOTAL:				

NOTES & MEAL IDEAS

MY KETO JOURNEY *Tracker*

SLEEP TRACKER: **DATE** _____

 RISE: _____   BEDTIME: _____   SLEEP (HRS): _____

NOTES FOR THE DAY

_____

_____

_____

EXERCISE / WORKOUT ROUTINE

TOP 6 PRIORITIES OF THE DAY

- ⦿ _____   ⦿ _____
- ⦿ _____   ⦿ _____
- ⦿ _____   ⦿ _____

IN A STATE OF KETOSIS?

YES   NO   UNSURE

WATER INTAKE TRACKER

💧 💧 💧 💧 💧 💧 💧 💧

DAILY ENERGY LEVEL

HIGH	**MEDIUM**	**LOW**

BREAKFAST

FAT: CARBS: PROTEIN: CALORIES:

LUNCH

FAT: CARBS: PROTEIN: CALORIES:

DINNER

FAT: CARBS: PROTEIN: CALORIES:

SNACKS

FAT: CARBS: PROTEIN: CALORIES:

END OF THE DAY TOTAL OVERVIEW

CARBS	FAT	PROTEIN	CALORIES

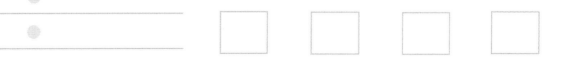

DAILY FOOD *Journal*

FOOD TRACKER

MEAL/SNACK	NET CARBS	FAT	CAL	PROTEIN
DAILY GOAL:			
TOTAL:			

NOTES & MEAL IDEAS

MY KETO JOURNEY *Tracker*

SLEEP TRACKER:

DATE _____

 | RISE: _____ | 🌙 | BEDTIME: _____ | 💤 | SLEEP (HRS): _____

NOTES FOR THE DAY

_____

_____

_____

EXERCISE / WORKOUT ROUTINE

TOP 6 PRIORITIES OF THE DAY

- ○ _____   ○ _____
- ○ _____   ○ _____
- ○ _____   ○ _____

IN A STATE OF KETOSIS?

YES   NO   UNSURE

WATER INTAKE TRACKER

💧 💧 💧 💧 💧 💧 💧 💧

DAILY ENERGY LEVEL

HIGH	MEDIUM	LOW

BREAKFAST

FAT: CARBS: PROTEIN: CALORIES:

LUNCH

FAT: CARBS: PROTEIN: CALORIES:

DINNER

FAT: CARBS: PROTEIN: CALORIES:

SNACKS

FAT: CARBS: PROTEIN: CALORIES:

END OF THE DAY TOTAL OVERVIEW

CARBS	FAT	PROTEIN	CALORIES

DAILY FOOD *Journal*

FOOD TRACKER

MEAL/SNACK	NET CARBS	FAT	CAL	PROTEIN
DAILY GOAL:				
TOTAL:				

NOTES & MEAL IDEAS

MY KETO JOURNEY *Tracker*

SLEEP TRACKER:

DATE _____

 RISE: [   ]   BEDTIME: [   ]   SLEEP (HRS): [   ]

NOTES FOR THE DAY

_____

_____

_____

EXERCISE / WORKOUT ROUTINE

TOP 6 PRIORITIES OF THE DAY

-
-
-
-
-
-

IN A STATE OF KETOSIS?

YES   NO   UNSURE

WATER INTAKE TRACKER

DAILY ENERGY LEVEL

HIGH   **MEDIUM**   **LOW**

BREAKFAST

FAT: CARBS: PROTEIN: CALORIES:

LUNCH

FAT: CARBS: PROTEIN: CALORIES:

DINNER

FAT: CARBS: PROTEIN: CALORIES:

SNACKS

FAT: CARBS: PROTEIN: CALORIES:

END OF THE DAY TOTAL OVERVIEW

CARBS	FAT	PROTEIN	CALORIES

DAILY FOOD *Journal*

FOOD TRACKER

MEAL/SNACK	NET CARBS	FAT	CAL	PROTEIN
DAILY GOAL:				
TOTAL:				

NOTES & MEAL IDEAS

MY KETO JOURNEY *Tracker*

SLEEP TRACKER:

DATE _____

 RISE: _____   BEDTIME: _____   SLEEP (HRS): _____

NOTES FOR THE DAY

_____
_____
_____

EXERCISE / WORKOUT ROUTINE

TOP 6 PRIORITIES OF THE DAY

IN A STATE OF KETOSIS?

YES   NO   UNSURE

WATER INTAKE TRACKER

DAILY ENERGY LEVEL

HIGH	MEDIUM	LOW

BREAKFAST

FAT: CARBS: PROTEIN: CALORIES:

LUNCH

FAT: CARBS: PROTEIN: CALORIES:

DINNER

FAT: CARBS: PROTEIN: CALORIES:

SNACKS

FAT: CARBS: PROTEIN: CALORIES:

END OF THE DAY TOTAL OVERVIEW

CARBS	FAT	PROTEIN	CALORIES

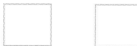
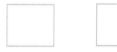

DAILY FOOD *Journal*

FOOD TRACKER

MEAL/SNACK	NET CARBS	FAT	CAL	PROTEIN
DAILY GOAL:				
TOTAL:				

NOTES & MEAL IDEAS

MY KETO JOURNEY *Tracker*

SLEEP TRACKER:

DATE _____

 | RISE: | | BEDTIME: | SLEEP (HRS):

NOTES FOR THE DAY

_____

_____

EXERCISE / WORKOUT ROUTINE

TOP 6 PRIORITIES OF THE DAY

- ○ _____   ○ _____
- ○ _____   ○ _____
- ○ _____   ○ _____

IN A STATE OF KETOSIS?

YES   NO   UNSURE

WATER INTAKE TRACKER

DAILY ENERGY LEVEL

HIGH	MEDIUM	LOW

BREAKFAST

FAT: CARBS: PROTEIN: CALORIES:

LUNCH

FAT: CARBS: PROTEIN: CALORIES:

DINNER

FAT: CARBS: PROTEIN: CALORIES:

SNACKS

FAT: CARBS: PROTEIN: CALORIES:

END OF THE DAY TOTAL OVERVIEW

CARBS	FAT	PROTEIN	CALORIES

DAILY FOOD *Journal*

FOOD TRACKER

MEAL/SNACK	NET CARBS	FAT	CAL	PROTEIN
DAILY GOAL:				
TOTAL:				

NOTES & MEAL IDEAS

MY KETO JOURNEY *Tracker*

SLEEP TRACKER:

DATE _____

 RISE: | BEDTIME: | SLEEP (HRS):

NOTES FOR THE DAY

_____

_____

_____

EXERCISE / WORKOUT ROUTINE

TOP 6 PRIORITIES OF THE DAY

- ● _____   ● _____
- ● _____   ● _____
- ● _____   ● _____

IN A STATE OF KETOSIS?

YES   NO   UNSURE

WATER INTAKE TRACKER

DAILY ENERGY LEVEL

HIGH   **MEDIUM**   **LOW**

BREAKFAST

FAT: CARBS: PROTEIN: CALORIES:

LUNCH

FAT: CARBS: PROTEIN: CALORIES:

DINNER

FAT: CARBS: PROTEIN: CALORIES:

SNACKS

FAT: CARBS: PROTEIN: CALORIES:

END OF THE DAY TOTAL OVERVIEW

CARBS	FAT	PROTEIN	CALORIES

DAILY FOOD *Journal*

FOOD TRACKER

MEAL/SNACK	NET CARBS	FAT	CAL	PROTEIN
DAILY GOAL:				
TOTAL:				

NOTES & MEAL IDEAS

MY KETO JOURNEY *Tracker*

SLEEP TRACKER:

DATE _____

 RISE: [   ]

BEDTIME: [   ]

 SLEEP (HRS): [   ]

NOTES FOR THE DAY

_____

_____

_____

EXERCISE / WORKOUT ROUTINE

[   ]

TOP 6 PRIORITIES OF THE DAY

- _____   - _____
- _____   - _____
- _____   - _____

IN A STATE OF KETOSIS?

YES   NO   UNSURE

WATER INTAKE TRACKER

DAILY ENERGY LEVEL

HIGH	**MEDIUM**	**LOW**

BREAKFAST

FAT: CARBS: PROTEIN: CALORIES:

LUNCH

FAT: CARBS: PROTEIN: CALORIES:

DINNER

FAT: CARBS: PROTEIN: CALORIES:

SNACKS

FAT: CARBS: PROTEIN: CALORIES:

END OF THE DAY TOTAL OVERVIEW

CARBS   FAT   PROTEIN   CALORIES

DAILY FOOD *Journal*

FOOD TRACKER

MEAL/SNACK	NET CARBS	FAT	CAL	PROTEIN
DAILY GOAL:				
TOTAL:				

NOTES & MEAL IDEAS

MY KETO JOURNEY *Tracker*

SLEEP TRACKER:

DATE _____

 RISE: | ☾ BEDTIME: | SLEEP (HRS):

NOTES FOR THE DAY

_____

_____

_____

EXERCISE / WORKOUT ROUTINE

TOP 6 PRIORITIES OF THE DAY

- ○ _____   ○ _____
- ○ _____   ○ _____
- ○ _____   ○ _____

IN A STATE OF KETOSIS?

YES   NO   UNSURE

WATER INTAKE TRACKER

💧 💧 💧 💧 💧 💧 💧 💧

DAILY ENERGY LEVEL		
HIGH	**MEDIUM**	**LOW**

BREAKFAST

FAT: CARBS: PROTEIN: CALORIES:

LUNCH

FAT: CARBS: PROTEIN: CALORIES:

DINNER

FAT: CARBS: PROTEIN: CALORIES:

SNACKS

FAT: CARBS: PROTEIN: CALORIES:

END OF THE DAY TOTAL OVERVIEW

CARBS	FAT	PROTEIN	CALORIES

DAILY FOOD *Journal*

FOOD TRACKER

MEAL/SNACK	NET CARBS	FAT	CAL	PROTEIN
DAILY GOAL:				
TOTAL:				

NOTES & MEAL IDEAS

MY KETO JOURNEY *Tracker*

SLEEP TRACKER:

DATE _____

 RISE: | BEDTIME: | SLEEP (HRS):

NOTES FOR THE DAY

_____
_____
_____

EXERCISE / WORKOUT ROUTINE

TOP 6 PRIORITIES OF THE DAY

- _____
- _____
- _____
- _____
- _____
- _____

IN A STATE OF KETOSIS?

YES   NO   UNSURE

WATER INTAKE TRACKER

DAILY ENERGY LEVEL

HIGH	MEDIUM	LOW

BREAKFAST

FAT: CARBS: PROTEIN: CALORIES:

LUNCH

FAT: CARBS: PROTEIN: CALORIES:

DINNER

FAT: CARBS: PROTEIN: CALORIES:

SNACKS

FAT: CARBS: PROTEIN: CALORIES:

END OF THE DAY TOTAL OVERVIEW

CARBS	FAT	PROTEIN	CALORIES

DAILY FOOD *Journal*

FOOD TRACKER

MEAL/SNACK	NET CARBS	FAT	CAL	PROTEIN
DAILY GOAL:				
TOTAL:				

NOTES & MEAL IDEAS

MY KETO JOURNEY *Tracker*

SLEEP TRACKER:

DATE _____

 RISE: _____

BEDTIME: _____

 SLEEP (HRS): _____

NOTES FOR THE DAY

_____

_____

_____

EXERCISE / WORKOUT ROUTINE

TOP 6 PRIORITIES OF THE DAY

- _____   - _____
- _____   - _____
- _____   - _____

IN A STATE OF KETOSIS?

YES   NO   UNSURE

WATER INTAKE TRACKER

DAILY ENERGY LEVEL

HIGH	MEDIUM	LOW

BREAKFAST

FAT: CARBS: PROTEIN: CALORIES:

LUNCH

FAT: CARBS: PROTEIN: CALORIES:

DINNER

FAT: CARBS: PROTEIN: CALORIES:

SNACKS

FAT: CARBS: PROTEIN: CALORIES:

END OF THE DAY TOTAL OVERVIEW

CARBS	FAT	PROTEIN	CALORIES

DAILY FOOD *Journal*

FOOD TRACKER

MEAL/SNACK	NET CARBS	FAT	CAL	PROTEIN
DAILY GOAL:				
TOTAL:				

NOTES & MEAL IDEAS

30-DAY
Progress

Weight and Measurements

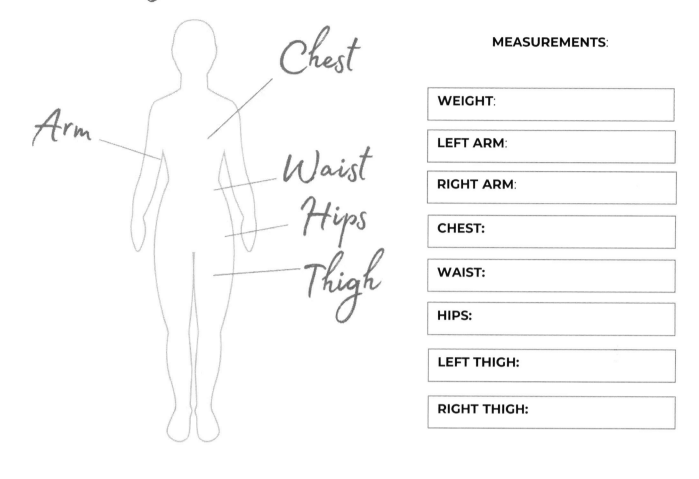

MEASUREMENTS:

WEIGHT:
LEFT ARM:
RIGHT ARM:
CHEST:
WAIST:
HIPS:
LEFT THIGH:
RIGHT THIGH:

My Journey

THOUGHTS ON MY PROGRESS:

MY KETO JOURNEY *Tracker*

SLEEP TRACKER:

 RISE: ___

BEDTIME: ___

 SLEEP (HRS): ___

DATE ___

NOTES FOR THE DAY

EXERCISE / WORKOUT ROUTINE

TOP 6 PRIORITIES OF THE DAY

- ○ ___
- ○ ___
- ○ ___
- ○ ___
- ○ ___
- ○ ___

IN A STATE OF KETOSIS?

YES   NO   UNSURE

WATER INTAKE TRACKER

DAILY ENERGY LEVEL

HIGH	MEDIUM	LOW

BREAKFAST

FAT: CARBS: PROTEIN: CALORIES:

LUNCH

FAT: CARBS: PROTEIN: CALORIES:

DINNER

FAT: CARBS: PROTEIN: CALORIES:

SNACKS

FAT: CARBS: PROTEIN: CALORIES:

END OF THE DAY TOTAL OVERVIEW

CARBS	FAT	PROTEIN	CALORIES

DAILY FOOD *Journal*

FOOD TRACKER

MEAL/SNACK	NET CARBS	FAT	CAL	PROTEIN
DAILY GOAL:				
TOTAL:				

NOTES & MEAL IDEAS

MY KETO JOURNEY *Tracker*

SLEEP TRACKER:

DATE _____

 RISE: _____   🌙 z z z BEDTIME: _____   SLEEP (HRS): _____

NOTES FOR THE DAY

_____

_____

_____

IN A STATE OF KETOSIS?

YES   NO   UNSURE

WATER INTAKE TRACKER

💧 💧 💧 💧 💧 💧 💧 💧

EXERCISE / WORKOUT ROUTINE

DAILY ENERGY LEVEL

HIGH	MEDIUM	LOW

BREAKFAST

FAT: CARBS: PROTEIN: CALORIES:

LUNCH

FAT: CARBS: PROTEIN: CALORIES:

DINNER

FAT: CARBS: PROTEIN: CALORIES:

SNACKS

FAT: CARBS: PROTEIN: CALORIES:

TOP 6 PRIORITIES OF THE DAY

● _____   ● _____

● _____   ● _____

● _____   ● _____

END OF THE DAY TOTAL OVERVIEW

CARBS	FAT	PROTEIN	CALORIES

DAILY FOOD *Journal*

FOOD TRACKER

MEAL/SNACK	NET CARBS	FAT	CAL	PROTEIN
DAILY GOAL:				
TOTAL:				

NOTES & MEAL IDEAS

MY KETO JOURNEY *Tracker*

SLEEP TRACKER:

DATE _____

 RISE: _____

🌙 BEDTIME: _____

 SLEEP (HRS): _____

NOTES FOR THE DAY

_____

_____

_____

EXERCISE / WORKOUT ROUTINE

TOP 6 PRIORITIES OF THE DAY

- ● _____   ● _____
- ● _____   ● _____
- ● _____   ● _____

IN A STATE OF KETOSIS?

YES   NO   UNSURE

WATER INTAKE TRACKER

💧 💧 💧 💧 💧 💧 💧 💧

DAILY ENERGY LEVEL

HIGH	MEDIUM	LOW

BREAKFAST

FAT: CARBS: PROTEIN: CALORIES:

LUNCH

FAT: CARBS: PROTEIN: CALORIES:

DINNER

FAT: CARBS: PROTEIN: CALORIES:

SNACKS

FAT: CARBS: PROTEIN: CALORIES:

END OF THE DAY TOTAL OVERVIEW

CARBS	FAT	PROTEIN	CALORIES

DAILY FOOD *Journal*

FOOD TRACKER

MEAL/SNACK	NET CARBS	FAT	CAL	PROTEIN
DAILY GOAL:				
TOTAL:				

NOTES & MEAL IDEAS

MY KETO JOURNEY *Tracker*

SLEEP TRACKER:

DATE _____

 RISE: _____   BEDTIME: _____   SLEEP (HRS): _____

NOTES FOR THE DAY

_____

_____

_____

EXERCISE / WORKOUT ROUTINE

TOP 6 PRIORITIES OF THE DAY

- ⦿ _____
- ⦿ _____
- ⦿ _____
- ⦿ _____
- ⦿ _____
- ⦿ _____

IN A STATE OF KETOSIS?

YES   NO   UNSURE

WATER INTAKE TRACKER

💧 💧 💧 💧 💧 💧 💧 💧

DAILY ENERGY LEVEL

HIGH   **MEDIUM**   **LOW**

BREAKFAST

FAT: CARBS: PROTEIN: CALORIES:

LUNCH

FAT: CARBS: PROTEIN: CALORIES:

DINNER

FAT: CARBS: PROTEIN: CALORIES:

SNACKS

FAT: CARBS: PROTEIN: CALORIES:

END OF THE DAY TOTAL OVERVIEW

CARBS   FAT   PROTEIN   CALORIES

DAILY FOOD *Journal*

FOOD TRACKER					NOTES & MEAL IDEAS
MEAL/SNACK	NET CARBS	FAT	CAL	PROTEIN	
DAILY GOAL:					
TOTAL:					

MY KETO JOURNEY *Tracker*

SLEEP TRACKER:

DATE _____

 RISE: _____   BEDTIME: _____   SLEEP (HRS): _____

NOTES FOR THE DAY

_____
_____
_____

EXERCISE / WORKOUT ROUTINE

TOP 6 PRIORITIES OF THE DAY

- ⚬ _____   ⚬ _____
- ⚬ _____   ⚬ _____
- ⚬ _____   ⚬ _____

IN A STATE OF KETOSIS?

YES   NO   UNSURE

WATER INTAKE TRACKER

DAILY ENERGY LEVEL

HIGH	MEDIUM	LOW

BREAKFAST

FAT: CARBS: PROTEIN: CALORIES:

LUNCH

FAT: CARBS: PROTEIN: CALORIES:

DINNER

FAT: CARBS: PROTEIN: CALORIES:

SNACKS

FAT: CARBS: PROTEIN: CALORIES:

END OF THE DAY TOTAL OVERVIEW

CARBS	FAT	PROTEIN	CALORIES

DAILY FOOD *Journal*

FOOD TRACKER

MEAL/SNACK	NET CARBS	FAT	CAL	PROTEIN
DAILY GOAL:				
TOTAL:				

NOTES & MEAL IDEAS

MY KETO JOURNEY *Tracker*

SLEEP TRACKER:

DATE _____

 RISE:

 BEDTIME:

 SLEEP (HRS):

NOTES FOR THE DAY

EXERCISE / WORKOUT ROUTINE

TOP 6 PRIORITIES OF THE DAY

- ⚪
- ⚪
- ⚪
- ⚪
- ⚪
- ⚪

IN A STATE OF KETOSIS?

YES   NO   UNSURE

WATER INTAKE TRACKER

DAILY ENERGY LEVEL		
HIGH	**MEDIUM**	**LOW**

BREAKFAST

FAT: CARBS: PROTEIN: CALORIES:

LUNCH

FAT: CARBS: PROTEIN: CALORIES:

DINNER

FAT: CARBS: PROTEIN: CALORIES:

SNACKS

FAT: CARBS: PROTEIN: CALORIES:

END OF THE DAY TOTAL OVERVIEW

CARBS	FAT	PROTEIN	CALORIES

DAILY FOOD *Journal*

FOOD TRACKER

MEAL/SNACK	NET CARBS	FAT	CAL	PROTEIN
DAILY GOAL:				
TOTAL:				

NOTES & MEAL IDEAS

MY KETO JOURNEY *Tracker*

SLEEP TRACKER:

DATE _____

 RISE: _____

BEDTIME: _____

 SLEEP (HRS): _____

NOTES FOR THE DAY

_____
_____
_____

EXERCISE / WORKOUT ROUTINE

TOP 6 PRIORITIES OF THE DAY

- _____ ● _____
- _____ ● _____
- _____ ● _____

IN A STATE OF KETOSIS?

YES   NO   UNSURE

WATER INTAKE TRACKER

DAILY ENERGY LEVEL

HIGH	MEDIUM	LOW

BREAKFAST

FAT: CARBS: PROTEIN: CALORIES:

LUNCH

FAT: CARBS: PROTEIN: CALORIES:

DINNER

FAT: CARBS: PROTEIN: CALORIES:

SNACKS

FAT: CARBS: PROTEIN: CALORIES:

END OF THE DAY TOTAL OVERVIEW

CARBS	FAT	PROTEIN	CALORIES

DAILY FOOD *Journal*

FOOD TRACKER

MEAL/SNACK	NET CARBS	FAT	CAL	PROTEIN
DAILY GOAL:				
TOTAL:				

NOTES & MEAL IDEAS

MY KETO JOURNEY *Tracker*

SLEEP TRACKER:

DATE _____

 | RISE: | BEDTIME: | SLEEP (HRS):

NOTES FOR THE DAY

_____
_____
_____

EXERCISE / WORKOUT ROUTINE

TOP 6 PRIORITIES OF THE DAY

- ● ●
- ● ●
- ● ●

IN A STATE OF KETOSIS?

YES   NO   UNSURE

WATER INTAKE TRACKER

DAILY ENERGY LEVEL

HIGH	MEDIUM	LOW

BREAKFAST

FAT: CARBS: PROTEIN: CALORIES:

LUNCH

FAT: CARBS: PROTEIN: CALORIES:

DINNER

FAT: CARBS: PROTEIN: CALORIES:

SNACKS

FAT: CARBS: PROTEIN: CALORIES:

END OF THE DAY TOTAL OVERVIEW

CARBS   FAT   PROTEIN   CALORIES

DAILY FOOD *Journal*

FOOD TRACKER

MEAL/SNACK	NET CARBS	FAT	CAL	PROTEIN
DAILY GOAL:				
TOTAL:				

NOTES & MEAL IDEAS

MY KETO JOURNEY *Tracker*

SLEEP TRACKER:

DATE _____

 RISE: | BEDTIME: | SLEEP (HRS):

NOTES FOR THE DAY

_____
_____
_____

EXERCISE / WORKOUT ROUTINE

TOP 6 PRIORITIES OF THE DAY

- _____   _____
- _____   _____
- _____   _____

IN A STATE OF KETOSIS?

YES   NO   UNSURE

WATER INTAKE TRACKER

DAILY ENERGY LEVEL

HIGH	**MEDIUM**	**LOW**

BREAKFAST

FAT: CARBS: PROTEIN: CALORIES:

LUNCH

FAT: CARBS: PROTEIN: CALORIES:

DINNER

FAT: CARBS: PROTEIN: CALORIES:

SNACKS

FAT: CARBS: PROTEIN: CALORIES:

END OF THE DAY TOTAL OVERVIEW

CARBS	FAT	PROTEIN	CALORIES

DAILY FOOD *Journal*

FOOD TRACKER

MEAL/SNACK	NET CARBS	FAT	CAL	PROTEIN
DAILY GOAL:				
TOTAL:				

NOTES & MEAL IDEAS

MY KETO JOURNEY *Tracker*

SLEEP TRACKER:

DATE _____

 RISE: | BEDTIME: | SLEEP (HRS):

NOTES FOR THE DAY

_____
_____
_____

EXERCISE / WORKOUT ROUTINE

TOP 6 PRIORITIES OF THE DAY

- ⬤
- ⬤
- ⬤
- ⬤
- ⬤
- ⬤

IN A STATE OF KETOSIS?

YES   NO   UNSURE

WATER INTAKE TRACKER

DAILY ENERGY LEVEL

HIGH	**MEDIUM**	**LOW**

BREAKFAST
FAT: CARBS: PROTEIN: CALORIES:

LUNCH
FAT: CARBS: PROTEIN: CALORIES:

DINNER
FAT: CARBS: PROTEIN: CALORIES:

SNACKS
FAT: CARBS: PROTEIN: CALORIES:

END OF THE DAY TOTAL OVERVIEW

CARBS	FAT	PROTEIN	CALORIES

DAILY FOOD *Journal*

FOOD TRACKER

MEAL/SNACK	NET CARBS	FAT	CAL	PROTEIN
DAILY GOAL:				
TOTAL:				

NOTES & MEAL IDEAS

MY KETO JOURNEY *Tracker*

SLEEP TRACKER:

DATE _____

 | RISE: | BEDTIME: | SLEEP (HRS):

NOTES FOR THE DAY

_____
_____
_____

EXERCISE / WORKOUT ROUTINE

TOP 6 PRIORITIES OF THE DAY

- _____   - _____
- _____   - _____
- _____   - _____

IN A STATE OF KETOSIS?

YES   NO   UNSURE

WATER INTAKE TRACKER

DAILY ENERGY LEVEL

HIGH	MEDIUM	LOW

BREAKFAST

FAT: CARBS: PROTEIN: CALORIES:

LUNCH

FAT: CARBS: PROTEIN: CALORIES:

DINNER

FAT: CARBS: PROTEIN: CALORIES:

SNACKS

FAT: CARBS: PROTEIN: CALORIES:

END OF THE DAY TOTAL OVERVIEW

CARBS	FAT	PROTEIN	CALORIES

DAILY FOOD *Journal*

MEAL/SNACK	NET CARBS	FAT	CAL	PROTEIN
DAILY GOAL:				
TOTAL:				

MY KETO JOURNEY *Tracker*

SLEEP TRACKER:

DATE _____

 RISE: | BEDTIME: | SLEEP (HRS):

NOTES FOR THE DAY

_____
_____
_____

EXERCISE / WORKOUT ROUTINE

TOP 6 PRIORITIES OF THE DAY

- ○ _____ ○ _____
- ○ _____ ○ _____
- ○ _____ ○ _____

IN A STATE OF KETOSIS?

YES   NO   UNSURE

WATER INTAKE TRACKER

DAILY ENERGY LEVEL

HIGH   **MEDIUM**   **LOW**

BREAKFAST

FAT: CARBS: PROTEIN: CALORIES:

LUNCH

FAT: CARBS: PROTEIN: CALORIES:

DINNER

FAT: CARBS: PROTEIN: CALORIES:

SNACKS

FAT: CARBS: PROTEIN: CALORIES:

END OF THE DAY TOTAL OVERVIEW

CARBS   FAT   PROTEIN   CALORIES

DAILY FOOD *Journal*

FOOD TRACKER

MEAL/SNACK	NET CARBS	FAT	CAL	PROTEIN
DAILY GOAL:				
TOTAL:				

MY KETO JOURNEY *Tracker*

SLEEP TRACKER:

DATE _____

 RISE: _____ 🌙 BEDTIME: _____ SLEEP (HRS): _____

NOTES FOR THE DAY

_____

_____

_____

EXERCISE / WORKOUT ROUTINE

TOP 6 PRIORITIES OF THE DAY

○ _____   ○ _____

○ _____   ○ _____

○ _____   ○ _____

IN A STATE OF KETOSIS?

YES   NO   UNSURE

WATER INTAKE TRACKER

💧 💧 💧 💧 💧 💧 💧 💧

DAILY ENERGY LEVEL		
HIGH	**MEDIUM**	**LOW**

BREAKFAST

FAT: CARBS: PROTEIN: CALORIES:

LUNCH

FAT: CARBS: PROTEIN: CALORIES:

DINNER

FAT: CARBS: PROTEIN: CALORIES:

SNACKS

FAT: CARBS: PROTEIN: CALORIES:

END OF THE DAY TOTAL OVERVIEW

CARBS	FAT	PROTEIN	CALORIES

DAILY FOOD *Journal*

FOOD TRACKER

MEAL/SNACK	NET CARBS	FAT	CAL	PROTEIN
DAILY GOAL:				
TOTAL:				

NOTES & MEAL IDEAS

MY KETO JOURNEY *Tracker*

SLEEP TRACKER:

DATE _____

 RISE: _____

 BEDTIME: _____

 SLEEP (HRS): _____

NOTES FOR THE DAY

_____

_____

_____

EXERCISE / WORKOUT ROUTINE

TOP 6 PRIORITIES OF THE DAY

- ⦿ _____ ⦿ _____
- ⦿ _____ ⦿ _____
- ⦿ _____ ⦿ _____

IN A STATE OF KETOSIS?

YES   NO   UNSURE

WATER INTAKE TRACKER

💧 💧 💧 💧 💧 💧 💧 💧

DAILY ENERGY LEVEL

HIGH   **MEDIUM**   **LOW**

BREAKFAST

FAT: CARBS: PROTEIN: CALORIES:

LUNCH

FAT: CARBS: PROTEIN: CALORIES:

DINNER

FAT: CARBS: PROTEIN: CALORIES:

SNACKS

FAT: CARBS: PROTEIN: CALORIES:

END OF THE DAY TOTAL OVERVIEW

CARBS   FAT   PROTEIN   CALORIES

DAILY FOOD *Journal*

FOOD TRACKER

MEAL/SNACK	NET CARBS	FAT	CAL	PROTEIN
DAILY GOAL:				
TOTAL:				

NOTES & MEAL IDEAS

MY KETO JOURNEY *Tracker*

SLEEP TRACKER:

DATE _____

 RISE: _____

🌙 BEDTIME: _____

 SLEEP (HRS): _____

NOTES FOR THE DAY

_____

_____

_____

EXERCISE / WORKOUT ROUTINE

TOP 6 PRIORITIES OF THE DAY

○ _____   ○ _____

○ _____   ○ _____

○ _____   ○ _____

IN A STATE OF KETOSIS?

YES   NO   UNSURE

WATER INTAKE TRACKER

💧 💧 💧 💧 💧 💧 💧 💧

DAILY ENERGY LEVEL

HIGH   **MEDIUM**   **LOW**

BREAKFAST

FAT: CARBS: PROTEIN: CALORIES:

LUNCH

FAT: CARBS: PROTEIN: CALORIES:

DINNER

FAT: CARBS: PROTEIN: CALORIES:

SNACKS

FAT: CARBS: PROTEIN: CALORIES:

END OF THE DAY TOTAL OVERVIEW

CARBS   FAT   PROTEIN   CALORIES

DAILY FOOD *Journal*

FOOD TRACKER					NOTES & MEAL IDEAS
MEAL/SNACK	NET CARBS	FAT	CAL	PROTEIN	
DAILY GOAL:					
TOTAL:					

MY KETO JOURNEY *Tracker*

SLEEP TRACKER:

DATE _____

 RISE: _____ BEDTIME: _____ SLEEP (HRS): _____

NOTES FOR THE DAY

_____

_____

_____

EXERCISE / WORKOUT ROUTINE

TOP 6 PRIORITIES OF THE DAY

- ○ _____   ○ _____
- ○ _____   ○ _____
- ○ _____   ○ _____

IN A STATE OF KETOSIS?

YES   NO   UNSURE

WATER INTAKE TRACKER

DAILY ENERGY LEVEL

HIGH	MEDIUM	LOW

BREAKFAST

FAT: CARBS: PROTEIN: CALORIES:

LUNCH

FAT: CARBS: PROTEIN: CALORIES:

DINNER

FAT: CARBS: PROTEIN: CALORIES:

SNACKS

FAT: CARBS: PROTEIN: CALORIES:

END OF THE DAY TOTAL OVERVIEW

CARBS	FAT	PROTEIN	CALORIES

DAILY FOOD *Journal*

FOOD TRACKER

MEAL/SNACK	NET CARBS	FAT	CAL	PROTEIN
DAILY GOAL:				
TOTAL:				

NOTES & MEAL IDEAS

MY KETO JOURNEY *Tracker*

SLEEP TRACKER:

DATE _____

 RISE: _____   🌙 BEDTIME: _____   SLEEP (HRS): _____

NOTES FOR THE DAY

_____
_____
_____

EXERCISE / WORKOUT ROUTINE

TOP 6 PRIORITIES OF THE DAY

⚬ _____   ⚬ _____
⚬ _____   ⚬ _____
⚬ _____   ⚬ _____

IN A STATE OF KETOSIS?

YES   NO   UNSURE

WATER INTAKE TRACKER

💧 💧 💧 💧 💧 💧 💧 💧

DAILY ENERGY LEVEL

HIGH	MEDIUM	LOW

BREAKFAST

FAT: CARBS: PROTEIN: CALORIES:

LUNCH

FAT: CARBS: PROTEIN: CALORIES:

DINNER

FAT: CARBS: PROTEIN: CALORIES:

SNACKS

FAT: CARBS: PROTEIN: CALORIES:

END OF THE DAY TOTAL OVERVIEW

CARBS	FAT	PROTEIN	CALORIES

DAILY FOOD *Journal*

FOOD TRACKER

MEAL/SNACK	NET CARBS	FAT	CAL	PROTEIN
DAILY GOAL:				
TOTAL:				

NOTES & MEAL IDEAS

MY KETO JOURNEY *Tracker*

SLEEP TRACKER:

DATE _____

| RISE: | BEDTIME: | SLEEP (HRS): |

NOTES FOR THE DAY

_____
_____
_____

EXERCISE / WORKOUT ROUTINE

TOP 6 PRIORITIES OF THE DAY

- ○ _____   ○ _____
- ○ _____   ○ _____
- ○ _____   ○ _____

IN A STATE OF KETOSIS?

YES   NO   UNSURE

WATER INTAKE TRACKER

DAILY ENERGY LEVEL

| **HIGH** | **MEDIUM** | **LOW** |

BREAKFAST

FAT: CARBS: PROTEIN: CALORIES:

LUNCH

FAT: CARBS: PROTEIN: CALORIES:

DINNER

FAT: CARBS: PROTEIN: CALORIES:

SNACKS

FAT: CARBS: PROTEIN: CALORIES:

END OF THE DAY TOTAL OVERVIEW

CARBS	FAT	PROTEIN	CALORIES

DAILY FOOD *Journal*

FOOD TRACKER				
MEAL/SNACK	NET CARBS	FAT	CAL	PROTEIN
DAILY GOAL:				
TOTAL:				

NOTES & MEAL IDEAS

MY KETO JOURNEY *Tracker*

SLEEP TRACKER:

DATE _____

 | RISE: _____ | | BEDTIME: _____ | | SLEEP (HRS): _____

NOTES FOR THE DAY

_____

_____

_____

EXERCISE / WORKOUT ROUTINE

TOP 6 PRIORITIES OF THE DAY

- ⚪ _____ ⚪ _____
- ⚪ _____ ⚪ _____
- ⚪ _____ ⚪ _____

IN A STATE OF KETOSIS?

YES   NO   UNSURE

WATER INTAKE TRACKER

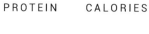

DAILY ENERGY LEVEL

HIGH   **MEDIUM**   **LOW**

BREAKFAST

FAT: CARBS: PROTEIN: CALORIES:

LUNCH

FAT: CARBS: PROTEIN: CALORIES:

DINNER

FAT: CARBS: PROTEIN: CALORIES:

SNACKS

FAT: CARBS: PROTEIN: CALORIES:

END OF THE DAY TOTAL OVERVIEW

CARBS   FAT   PROTEIN   CALORIES

 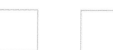

DAILY FOOD *Journal*

FOOD TRACKER

MEAL/SNACK	NET CARBS	FAT	CAL	PROTEIN
DAILY GOAL:				
TOTAL:				

NOTES & MEAL IDEAS

MY KETO JOURNEY *Tracker*

SLEEP TRACKER:

DATE _____

 | RISE: | | BEDTIME: | | SLEEP (HRS): |

NOTES FOR THE DAY

_____

_____

_____

IN A STATE OF KETOSIS?

YES   NO   UNSURE

WATER INTAKE TRACKER

EXERCISE / WORKOUT ROUTINE

DAILY ENERGY LEVEL

HIGH	MEDIUM	LOW

BREAKFAST

FAT: CARBS: PROTEIN: CALORIES:

LUNCH

FAT: CARBS: PROTEIN: CALORIES:

DINNER

FAT: CARBS: PROTEIN: CALORIES:

SNACKS

FAT: CARBS: PROTEIN: CALORIES:

TOP 6 PRIORITIES OF THE DAY

END OF THE DAY TOTAL OVERVIEW

CARBS	FAT	PROTEIN	CALORIES

DAILY FOOD *Journal*

FOOD TRACKER

MEAL/SNACK	NET CARBS	FAT	CAL	PROTEIN
DAILY GOAL:				
TOTAL:				

NOTES & MEAL IDEAS

MY KETO JOURNEY *Tracker*

SLEEP TRACKER:

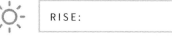 RISE: _____

 BEDTIME: _____

 SLEEP (HRS): _____

DATE _____

NOTES FOR THE DAY

_____

_____

_____

EXERCISE / WORKOUT ROUTINE

TOP 6 PRIORITIES OF THE DAY

- _____ - _____
- _____ - _____
- _____ - _____

IN A STATE OF KETOSIS?

YES   NO   UNSURE

WATER INTAKE TRACKER

DAILY ENERGY LEVEL

HIGH	**MEDIUM**	**LOW**

BREAKFAST

FAT: CARBS: PROTEIN: CALORIES:

LUNCH

FAT: CARBS: PROTEIN: CALORIES:

DINNER

FAT: CARBS: PROTEIN: CALORIES:

SNACKS

FAT: CARBS: PROTEIN: CALORIES:

END OF THE DAY TOTAL OVERVIEW

CARBS	FAT	PROTEIN	CALORIES

DAILY FOOD *Journal*

FOOD TRACKER

MEAL/SNACK	NET CARBS	FAT	CAL	PROTEIN
DAILY GOAL:				
TOTAL:				

NOTES & MEAL IDEAS

MY KETO JOURNEY *Tracker*

SLEEP TRACKER:

DATE _____

 RISE: _____   🌙 zzz BEDTIME: _____   💭zᶻZ SLEEP (HRS): _____

NOTES FOR THE DAY

_____

_____

_____

EXERCISE / WORKOUT ROUTINE

IN A STATE OF KETOSIS?

YES   NO   UNSURE

WATER INTAKE TRACKER

💧 💧 💧 💧 💧 💧 💧 💧

DAILY ENERGY LEVEL

HIGH	**MEDIUM**	**LOW**

BREAKFAST

FAT: CARBS: PROTEIN: CALORIES:

LUNCH

FAT: CARBS: PROTEIN: CALORIES:

DINNER

FAT: CARBS: PROTEIN: CALORIES:

SNACKS

FAT: CARBS: PROTEIN: CALORIES:

TOP 6 PRIORITIES OF THE DAY

● _____   ● _____

● _____   ● _____

● _____   ● _____

END OF THE DAY TOTAL OVERVIEW

CARBS	FAT	PROTEIN	CALORIES

DAILY FOOD *Journal*

FOOD TRACKER

MEAL/SNACK	NET CARBS	FAT	CAL	PROTEIN
DAILY GOAL:				
TOTAL:				

NOTES & MEAL IDEAS

MY KETO JOURNEY *Tracker*

SLEEP TRACKER:

DATE _____

 RISE: _____

🌙 BEDTIME: _____

 SLEEP (HRS): _____

NOTES FOR THE DAY

_____
_____
_____

IN A STATE OF KETOSIS?

YES   NO   UNSURE

WATER INTAKE TRACKER

EXERCISE / WORKOUT ROUTINE

DAILY ENERGY LEVEL		
HIGH	**MEDIUM**	**LOW**

BREAKFAST

FAT: CARBS: PROTEIN: CALORIES:

LUNCH

FAT: CARBS: PROTEIN: CALORIES:

DINNER

FAT: CARBS: PROTEIN: CALORIES:

SNACKS

FAT: CARBS: PROTEIN: CALORIES:

TOP 6 PRIORITIES OF THE DAY

- _____
- _____
- _____
- _____
- _____
- _____

END OF THE DAY TOTAL OVERVIEW

CARBS	FAT	PROTEIN	CALORIES

DAILY FOOD *Journal*

FOOD TRACKER

MEAL/SNACK	NET CARBS	FAT	CAL	PROTEIN
DAILY GOAL:				
TOTAL:				

NOTES & MEAL IDEAS

MY KETO JOURNEY *Tracker*

SLEEP TRACKER:

DATE _____

☀ | RISE: | | BEDTIME: | | SLEEP (HRS):

NOTES FOR THE DAY

_____
_____
_____

EXERCISE / WORKOUT ROUTINE

TOP 6 PRIORITIES OF THE DAY

● _____ ● _____
● _____ ● _____
● _____ ● _____

IN A STATE OF KETOSIS?

YES   NO   UNSURE

WATER INTAKE TRACKER

DAILY ENERGY LEVEL

HIGH	**MEDIUM**	**LOW**

BREAKFAST

FAT: CARBS: PROTEIN: CALORIES:

LUNCH

FAT: CARBS: PROTEIN: CALORIES:

DINNER

FAT: CARBS: PROTEIN: CALORIES:

SNACKS

FAT: CARBS: PROTEIN: CALORIES:

END OF THE DAY TOTAL OVERVIEW

CARBS	FAT	PROTEIN	CALORIES

DAILY FOOD *Journal*

FOOD TRACKER

MEAL/SNACK	NET CARBS	FAT	CAL	PROTEIN
DAILY GOAL:				
TOTAL:				

NOTES & MEAL IDEAS

MY KETO JOURNEY *Tracker*

SLEEP TRACKER:

DATE _____

☀ RISE: | 🌙 BEDTIME: | 💤 SLEEP (HRS):

NOTES FOR THE DAY

_____
_____
_____

IN A STATE OF KETOSIS?

YES   NO   UNSURE

WATER INTAKE TRACKER

💧 💧 💧 💧 💧 💧 💧 💧

EXERCISE / WORKOUT ROUTINE

DAILY ENERGY LEVEL

HIGH   **MEDIUM**   **LOW**

BREAKFAST

FAT: CARBS: PROTEIN: CALORIES:

LUNCH

FAT: CARBS: PROTEIN: CALORIES:

DINNER

FAT: CARBS: PROTEIN: CALORIES:

SNACKS

FAT: CARBS: PROTEIN: CALORIES:

TOP 6 PRIORITIES OF THE DAY

- _____   - _____
- _____   - _____
- _____   - _____

END OF THE DAY TOTAL OVERVIEW

CARBS   FAT   PROTEIN   CALORIES

DAILY FOOD *Journal*

FOOD TRACKER

MEAL/SNACK	NET CARBS	FAT	CAL	PROTEIN
DAILY GOAL:				
TOTAL:				

NOTES & MEAL IDEAS

MY KETO JOURNEY *Tracker*

SLEEP TRACKER:

DATE _____

☼ | RISE: | | BEDTIME: | | SLEEP (HRS):

NOTES FOR THE DAY

_____
_____
_____

EXERCISE / WORKOUT ROUTINE

IN A STATE OF KETOSIS?

YES   NO   UNSURE

WATER INTAKE TRACKER

💧 💧 💧 💧 💧 💧 💧 💧

DAILY ENERGY LEVEL		
HIGH	**MEDIUM**	**LOW**

BREAKFAST

FAT: CARBS: PROTEIN: CALORIES:

LUNCH

FAT: CARBS: PROTEIN: CALORIES:

DINNER

FAT: CARBS: PROTEIN: CALORIES:

SNACKS

FAT: CARBS: PROTEIN: CALORIES:

TOP 6 PRIORITIES OF THE DAY

● _____   ● _____
● _____   ● _____
● _____   ● _____

END OF THE DAY TOTAL OVERVIEW

CARBS   FAT   PROTEIN   CALORIES

☐   ☐   ☐   ☐

DAILY FOOD *Journal*

FOOD TRACKER

MEAL/SNACK	NET CARBS	FAT	CAL	PROTEIN
DAILY GOAL:				
TOTAL:				

NOTES & MEAL IDEAS

MY KETO JOURNEY *Tracker*

SLEEP TRACKER:

DATE _____

RISE:	BEDTIME:	SLEEP (HRS):

NOTES FOR THE DAY

_____
_____
_____

EXERCISE / WORKOUT ROUTINE

TOP 6 PRIORITIES OF THE DAY

- ○ _____   ○ _____
- ○ _____   ○ _____
- ○ _____   ○ _____

IN A STATE OF KETOSIS?

YES   NO   UNSURE

WATER INTAKE TRACKER

DAILY ENERGY LEVEL

HIGH	MEDIUM	LOW

BREAKFAST

FAT: CARBS: PROTEIN: CALORIES:

LUNCH

FAT: CARBS: PROTEIN: CALORIES:

DINNER

FAT: CARBS: PROTEIN: CALORIES:

SNACKS

FAT: CARBS: PROTEIN: CALORIES:

END OF THE DAY TOTAL OVERVIEW

CARBS	FAT	PROTEIN	CALORIES

DAILY FOOD *Journal*

FOOD TRACKER

MEAL/SNACK	NET CARBS	FAT	CAL	PROTEIN
DAILY GOAL:				
TOTAL:				

NOTES & MEAL IDEAS

MY KETO JOURNEY *Tracker*

SLEEP TRACKER:

DATE _____

 RISE: [   ]   🌙 BEDTIME: [   ]   SLEEP (HRS): [   ]

NOTES FOR THE DAY	IN A STATE OF KETOSIS?

_____

_____

_____

YES   NO   UNSURE

WATER INTAKE TRACKER

💧 💧 💧 💧 💧 💧 💧 💧

EXERCISE / WORKOUT ROUTINE

DAILY ENERGY LEVEL		
HIGH	**MEDIUM**	**LOW**

BREAKFAST

FAT: CARBS: PROTEIN: CALORIES:

LUNCH

FAT: CARBS: PROTEIN: CALORIES:

DINNER

FAT: CARBS: PROTEIN: CALORIES:

SNACKS

FAT: CARBS: PROTEIN: CALORIES:

TOP 6 PRIORITIES OF THE DAY

- _____   - _____
- _____   - _____
- _____   - _____

END OF THE DAY TOTAL OVERVIEW

CARBS	FAT	PROTEIN	CALORIES
_____	_____	_____	_____
[ ]	[ ]	[ ]	[ ]

DAILY FOOD *Journal*

FOOD TRACKER

MEAL/SNACK	NET CARBS	FAT	CAL	PROTEIN
DAILY GOAL:				
TOTAL:				

NOTES & MEAL IDEAS

MY KETO JOURNEY *Tracker*

SLEEP TRACKER:

DATE _____

☀ | RISE: | 🌙 zzz | BEDTIME: | 💭zᶻᶻ | SLEEP (HRS):

NOTES FOR THE DAY

_____

_____

_____

EXERCISE / WORKOUT ROUTINE

TOP 6 PRIORITIES OF THE DAY

● _____ ● _____

● _____ ● _____

● _____ ● _____

IN A STATE OF KETOSIS?

YES   NO   UNSURE

WATER INTAKE TRACKER

💧 💧 💧 💧 💧 💧 💧

DAILY ENERGY LEVEL

HIGH	**MEDIUM**	**LOW**

BREAKFAST

FAT: CARBS: PROTEIN: CALORIES:

LUNCH

FAT: CARBS: PROTEIN: CALORIES:

DINNER

FAT: CARBS: PROTEIN: CALORIES:

SNACKS

FAT: CARBS: PROTEIN: CALORIES:

END OF THE DAY TOTAL OVERVIEW

CARBS	FAT	PROTEIN	CALORIES

DAILY FOOD *Journal*

FOOD TRACKER

MEAL/SNACK	NET CARBS	FAT	CAL	PROTEIN
DAILY GOAL:				
TOTAL:				

NOTES & MEAL IDEAS

MY KETO JOURNEY *Tracker*

SLEEP TRACKER:

DATE _____

| | RISE: | | BEDTIME: | | SLEEP (HRS): |

NOTES FOR THE DAY

_____

_____

_____

EXERCISE / WORKOUT ROUTINE

TOP 6 PRIORITIES OF THE DAY

- ●
- ●
- ●
- ●
- ●
- ●

IN A STATE OF KETOSIS?

YES   NO   UNSURE

WATER INTAKE TRACKER

DAILY ENERGY LEVEL

| **HIGH** | **MEDIUM** | **LOW** |

BREAKFAST

FAT: CARBS: PROTEIN: CALORIES:

LUNCH

FAT: CARBS: PROTEIN: CALORIES:

DINNER

FAT: CARBS: PROTEIN: CALORIES:

SNACKS

FAT: CARBS: PROTEIN: CALORIES:

END OF THE DAY TOTAL OVERVIEW

CARBS	FAT	PROTEIN	CALORIES

DAILY FOOD *Journal*

FOOD TRACKER

MEAL/SNACK	NET CARBS	FAT	CAL	PROTEIN
DAILY GOAL:				
TOTAL:				

NOTES & MEAL IDEAS

60-DAY
Progress

Weight and Measurements

Chest

Arm

Waist

Hips

Thigh

MEASUREMENTS:

WEIGHT:

LEFT ARM:

RIGHT ARM:

CHEST:

WAIST:

HIPS:

LEFT THIGH:

RIGHT THIGH:

My Journey

THOUGHTS ON MY PROGRESS:

MY KETO JOURNEY *Tracker*

SLEEP TRACKER:

DATE _____

RISE: _____   BEDTIME: _____   SLEEP (HRS): _____

NOTES FOR THE DAY

_____

_____

_____

IN A STATE OF KETOSIS?

YES   NO   UNSURE

WATER INTAKE TRACKER

EXERCISE / WORKOUT ROUTINE

DAILY ENERGY LEVEL		
HIGH	**MEDIUM**	**LOW**

BREAKFAST

FAT: CARBS: PROTEIN: CALORIES:

LUNCH

FAT: CARBS: PROTEIN: CALORIES:

DINNER

FAT: CARBS: PROTEIN: CALORIES:

SNACKS

FAT: CARBS: PROTEIN: CALORIES:

TOP 6 PRIORITIES OF THE DAY

END OF THE DAY TOTAL OVERVIEW

CARBS	FAT	PROTEIN	CALORIES

DAILY FOOD *Journal*

FOOD TRACKER

MEAL/SNACK	NET CARBS	FAT	CAL	PROTEIN
DAILY GOAL:				
TOTAL:				

NOTES & MEAL IDEAS

MY KETO JOURNEY *Tracker*

SLEEP TRACKER:

DATE _____

 RISE: [   ]   🌙 BEDTIME: [   ]   SLEEP (HRS): [   ]

NOTES FOR THE DAY

_____

_____

_____

EXERCISE / WORKOUT ROUTINE

TOP 6 PRIORITIES OF THE DAY

- ● _____   ● _____
- ● _____   ● _____
- ● _____   ● _____

IN A STATE OF KETOSIS?

YES   NO   UNSURE

WATER INTAKE TRACKER

💧 💧 💧 💧 💧 💧 💧

DAILY ENERGY LEVEL

HIGH   **MEDIUM**   **LOW**

BREAKFAST

FAT: CARBS: PROTEIN: CALORIES:

LUNCH

FAT: CARBS: PROTEIN: CALORIES:

DINNER

FAT: CARBS: PROTEIN: CALORIES:

SNACKS

FAT: CARBS: PROTEIN: CALORIES:

END OF THE DAY TOTAL OVERVIEW

CARBS	FAT	PROTEIN	CALORIES
[ ]	[ ]	[ ]	[ ]

DAILY FOOD *Journal*

FOOD TRACKER

MEAL/SNACK	NET CARBS	FAT	CAL	PROTEIN
DAILY GOAL:				
TOTAL:				

NOTES & MEAL IDEAS

MY KETO JOURNEY *Tracker*

SLEEP TRACKER:

DATE _____

 RISE:

BEDTIME:

 SLEEP (HRS):

NOTES FOR THE DAY

_____

_____

_____

EXERCISE / WORKOUT ROUTINE

TOP 6 PRIORITIES OF THE DAY

• _____   • _____

• _____   • _____

• _____   • _____

IN A STATE OF KETOSIS?

YES   NO   UNSURE

WATER INTAKE TRACKER

DAILY ENERGY LEVEL		
HIGH	**MEDIUM**	**LOW**

BREAKFAST

FAT: CARBS: PROTEIN: CALORIES:

LUNCH

FAT: CARBS: PROTEIN: CALORIES:

DINNER

FAT: CARBS: PROTEIN: CALORIES:

SNACKS

FAT: CARBS: PROTEIN: CALORIES:

END OF THE DAY TOTAL OVERVIEW

CARBS	FAT	PROTEIN	CALORIES

DAILY FOOD *Journal*

FOOD TRACKER

MEAL/SNACK	NET CARBS	FAT	CAL	PROTEIN
DAILY GOAL:				
TOTAL:				

NOTES & MEAL IDEAS

MY KETO JOURNEY *Tracker*

SLEEP TRACKER:

DATE _____

 RISE: _____

🌙 BEDTIME: _____

💤 SLEEP (HRS): _____

NOTES FOR THE DAY

_____

_____

_____

EXERCISE / WORKOUT ROUTINE

TOP 6 PRIORITIES OF THE DAY

- ⚫ _____   ⚫ _____
- ⚫ _____   ⚫ _____
- ⚫ _____   ⚫ _____

IN A STATE OF KETOSIS?

YES   NO   UNSURE

WATER INTAKE TRACKER

💧 💧 💧 💧 💧 💧 💧 💧

DAILY ENERGY LEVEL

HIGH	**MEDIUM**	**LOW**

BREAKFAST

FAT: CARBS: PROTEIN: CALORIES:

LUNCH

FAT: CARBS: PROTEIN: CALORIES:

DINNER

FAT: CARBS: PROTEIN: CALORIES:

SNACKS

FAT: CARBS: PROTEIN: CALORIES:

END OF THE DAY TOTAL OVERVIEW

CARBS	FAT	PROTEIN	CALORIES

DAILY FOOD *Journal*

FOOD TRACKER

MEAL/SNACK	NET CARBS	FAT	CAL	PROTEIN
DAILY GOAL:				
TOTAL:				

NOTES & MEAL IDEAS

MY KETO JOURNEY *Tracker*

SLEEP TRACKER:

DATE _____

RISE: | BEDTIME: | SLEEP (HRS):

NOTES FOR THE DAY

EXERCISE / WORKOUT ROUTINE

IN A STATE OF KETOSIS?

YES   NO   UNSURE

WATER INTAKE TRACKER

DAILY ENERGY LEVEL

HIGH	MEDIUM	LOW

BREAKFAST

FAT: CARBS: PROTEIN: CALORIES:

LUNCH

FAT: CARBS: PROTEIN: CALORIES:

DINNER

FAT: CARBS: PROTEIN: CALORIES:

SNACKS

FAT: CARBS: PROTEIN: CALORIES:

TOP 6 PRIORITIES OF THE DAY

END OF THE DAY TOTAL OVERVIEW

CARBS	FAT	PROTEIN	CALORIES

DAILY FOOD *Journal*

FOOD TRACKER

MEAL/SNACK	NET CARBS	FAT	CAL	PROTEIN
DAILY GOAL:				
TOTAL:				

NOTES & MEAL IDEAS

MY KETO JOURNEY *Tracker*

SLEEP TRACKER:

DATE _____

 RISE: _____

BEDTIME: _____

 SLEEP (HRS): _____

NOTES FOR THE DAY

_____
_____
_____

IN A STATE OF KETOSIS?

YES   NO   UNSURE

WATER INTAKE TRACKER

EXERCISE / WORKOUT ROUTINE

DAILY ENERGY LEVEL		
HIGH	**MEDIUM**	**LOW**

BREAKFAST

FAT: CARBS: PROTEIN: CALORIES:

LUNCH

FAT: CARBS: PROTEIN: CALORIES:

DINNER

FAT: CARBS: PROTEIN: CALORIES:

SNACKS

FAT: CARBS: PROTEIN: CALORIES:

TOP 6 PRIORITIES OF THE DAY

END OF THE DAY TOTAL OVERVIEW

CARBS	FAT	PROTEIN	CALORIES

DAILY FOOD *Journal*

FOOD TRACKER

MEAL/SNACK	NET CARBS	FAT	CAL	PROTEIN
DAILY GOAL:				
TOTAL:				

NOTES & MEAL IDEAS

MY KETO JOURNEY *Tracker*

SLEEP TRACKER:

DATE _____

RISE:		BEDTIME:		SLEEP (HRS):

NOTES FOR THE DAY

_____

_____

_____

EXERCISE / WORKOUT ROUTINE

IN A STATE OF KETOSIS?

YES   NO   UNSURE

WATER INTAKE TRACKER

DAILY ENERGY LEVEL

HIGH	MEDIUM	LOW

BREAKFAST

FAT: CARBS: PROTEIN: CALORIES:

LUNCH

FAT: CARBS: PROTEIN: CALORIES:

DINNER

FAT: CARBS: PROTEIN: CALORIES:

SNACKS

FAT: CARBS: PROTEIN: CALORIES:

TOP 6 PRIORITIES OF THE DAY

- _____
- _____
- _____
- _____
- _____
- _____

END OF THE DAY TOTAL OVERVIEW

CARBS	FAT	PROTEIN	CALORIES

DAILY FOOD *Journal*

FOOD TRACKER

MEAL/SNACK	NET CARBS	FAT	CAL	PROTEIN
DAILY GOAL:				
TOTAL:				

NOTES & MEAL IDEAS

MY KETO JOURNEY *Tracker*

SLEEP TRACKER:

DATE _____

| RISE: | BEDTIME: | SLEEP (HRS): |

NOTES FOR THE DAY

....

....

....

EXERCISE / WORKOUT ROUTINE

IN A STATE OF KETOSIS?

YES   NO   UNSURE

WATER INTAKE TRACKER

DAILY ENERGY LEVEL

| HIGH | MEDIUM | LOW |

BREAKFAST

FAT: CARBS: PROTEIN: CALORIES:

LUNCH

FAT: CARBS: PROTEIN: CALORIES:

DINNER

FAT: CARBS: PROTEIN: CALORIES:

SNACKS

FAT: CARBS: PROTEIN: CALORIES:

TOP 6 PRIORITIES OF THE DAY

END OF THE DAY TOTAL OVERVIEW

| CARBS | FAT | PROTEIN | CALORIES |

DAILY FOOD *Journal*

FOOD TRACKER

MEAL/SNACK	NET CARBS	FAT	CAL	PROTEIN
DAILY GOAL:				
TOTAL:				

NOTES & MEAL IDEAS

MY KETO JOURNEY *Tracker*

SLEEP TRACKER:

DATE _____

RISE: [ ]   BEDTIME: [ ]   SLEEP (HRS): [ ]

NOTES FOR THE DAY

_____
_____
_____

EXERCISE / WORKOUT ROUTINE

TOP 6 PRIORITIES OF THE DAY

- ● _____
- ● _____
- ● _____
- ● _____
- ● _____
- ● _____

IN A STATE OF KETOSIS?

YES   NO   UNSURE

WATER INTAKE TRACKER

💧 💧 💧 💧 💧 💧 💧 💧

DAILY ENERGY LEVEL

HIGH	MEDIUM	LOW

BREAKFAST

FAT: CARBS: PROTEIN: CALORIES:

LUNCH

FAT: CARBS: PROTEIN: CALORIES:

DINNER

FAT: CARBS: PROTEIN: CALORIES:

SNACKS

FAT: CARBS: PROTEIN: CALORIES:

END OF THE DAY TOTAL OVERVIEW

CARBS	FAT	PROTEIN	CALORIES
_____	_____	_____	_____
[ ]	[ ]	[ ]	[ ]

DAILY FOOD *Journal*

FOOD TRACKER

MEAL/SNACK	NET CARBS	FAT	CAL	PROTEIN
DAILY GOAL:				
TOTAL:				

NOTES & MEAL IDEAS

MY KETO JOURNEY *Tracker*

SLEEP TRACKER:

DATE _____

 RISE: _____   ☾ BEDTIME: _____   SLEEP (HRS): _____

NOTES FOR THE DAY

_____
_____
_____

EXERCISE / WORKOUT ROUTINE

TOP 6 PRIORITIES OF THE DAY

- _____   - _____
- _____   - _____
- _____   - _____

IN A STATE OF KETOSIS?

YES   NO   UNSURE

WATER INTAKE TRACKER

DAILY ENERGY LEVEL

HIGH	MEDIUM	LOW

BREAKFAST

FAT: CARBS: PROTEIN: CALORIES:

LUNCH

FAT: CARBS: PROTEIN: CALORIES:

DINNER

FAT: CARBS: PROTEIN: CALORIES:

SNACKS

FAT: CARBS: PROTEIN: CALORIES:

END OF THE DAY TOTAL OVERVIEW

CARBS	FAT	PROTEIN	CALORIES

DAILY FOOD *Journal*

FOOD TRACKER

MEAL/SNACK	NET CARBS	FAT	CAL	PROTEIN
DAILY GOAL:				
TOTAL:				

NOTES & MEAL IDEAS

MY KETO JOURNEY *Tracker*

SLEEP TRACKER:

DATE _____

☀ | RISE: | 🌙 zzz | BEDTIME: | ☁zzz | SLEEP (HRS):

NOTES FOR THE DAY

_____
_____
_____

IN A STATE OF KETOSIS?

YES   NO   UNSURE

WATER INTAKE TRACKER

💧 💧 💧 💧 💧 💧 💧 💧

EXERCISE / WORKOUT ROUTINE

DAILY ENERGY LEVEL		
HIGH	**MEDIUM**	**LOW**

BREAKFAST

FAT: CARBS: PROTEIN: CALORIES:

LUNCH

FAT: CARBS: PROTEIN: CALORIES:

DINNER

FAT: CARBS: PROTEIN: CALORIES:

SNACKS

FAT: CARBS: PROTEIN: CALORIES:

TOP 6 PRIORITIES OF THE DAY

● _____   ● _____
● _____   ● _____
● _____   ● _____

END OF THE DAY TOTAL OVERVIEW

CARBS   FAT   PROTEIN   CALORIES

DAILY FOOD *Journal*

FOOD TRACKER

MEAL/SNACK	NET CARBS	FAT	CAL	PROTEIN
DAILY GOAL:				
TOTAL:				

NOTES & MEAL IDEAS

MY KETO JOURNEY *Tracker*

SLEEP TRACKER:

DATE _____

☀ | RISE: | 🌙 zzz | BEDTIME: | 💭zzz | SLEEP (HRS):

NOTES FOR THE DAY

_____
_____
_____

EXERCISE / WORKOUT ROUTINE

TOP 6 PRIORITIES OF THE DAY

● _____   ● _____

● _____   ● _____

● _____   ● _____

IN A STATE OF KETOSIS?

YES   NO   UNSURE

WATER INTAKE TRACKER

💧 💧 💧 💧 💧 💧 💧 💧

DAILY ENERGY LEVEL

HIGH	**MEDIUM**	**LOW**

BREAKFAST

FAT: CARBS: PROTEIN: CALORIES:

LUNCH

FAT: CARBS: PROTEIN: CALORIES:

DINNER

FAT: CARBS: PROTEIN: CALORIES:

SNACKS

FAT: CARBS: PROTEIN: CALORIES:

END OF THE DAY TOTAL OVERVIEW

CARBS   FAT   PROTEIN   CALORIES

_____   _____   _____   _____

DAILY FOOD *Journal*

FOOD TRACKER					NOTES & MEAL IDEAS
MEAL/SNACK	NET CARBS	FAT	CAL	PROTEIN	
DAILY GOAL:					
TOTAL:					

MY KETO JOURNEY *Tracker*

SLEEP TRACKER:

DATE _____

 RISE: _____   BEDTIME: _____   SLEEP (HRS): _____

NOTES FOR THE DAY

_____
_____
_____

EXERCISE / WORKOUT ROUTINE

TOP 6 PRIORITIES OF THE DAY

- _____   - _____
- _____   - _____
- _____   - _____

IN A STATE OF KETOSIS?

YES   NO   UNSURE

WATER INTAKE TRACKER

DAILY ENERGY LEVEL

HIGH	MEDIUM	LOW

BREAKFAST

FAT: CARBS: PROTEIN: CALORIES:

LUNCH

FAT: CARBS: PROTEIN: CALORIES:

DINNER

FAT: CARBS: PROTEIN: CALORIES:

SNACKS

FAT: CARBS: PROTEIN: CALORIES:

END OF THE DAY TOTAL OVERVIEW

CARBS	FAT	PROTEIN	CALORIES

DAILY FOOD *Journal*

FOOD TRACKER

MEAL/SNACK	NET CARBS	FAT	CAL	PROTEIN
DAILY GOAL:				
TOTAL:				

NOTES & MEAL IDEAS

MY KETO JOURNEY *Tracker*

SLEEP TRACKER:

DATE _____

 RISE: _____

🌙 BEDTIME: _____

 SLEEP (HRS): _____

NOTES FOR THE DAY

_____

_____

_____

EXERCISE / WORKOUT ROUTINE

TOP 6 PRIORITIES OF THE DAY

● _____   ● _____

● _____   ● _____

● _____   ● _____

IN A STATE OF KETOSIS?

YES   NO   UNSURE

WATER INTAKE TRACKER

💧 💧 💧 💧 💧 💧 💧 💧

DAILY ENERGY LEVEL

HIGH	MEDIUM	LOW

BREAKFAST

FAT: CARBS: PROTEIN: CALORIES:

LUNCH

FAT: CARBS: PROTEIN: CALORIES:

DINNER

FAT: CARBS: PROTEIN: CALORIES:

SNACKS

FAT: CARBS: PROTEIN: CALORIES:

END OF THE DAY TOTAL OVERVIEW

CARBS	FAT	PROTEIN	CALORIES

DAILY FOOD *Journal*

<table>
<tr><td colspan="5">**FOOD TRACKER**</td><td>**NOTES & MEAL IDEAS**</td></tr>
<tr><td>MEAL/SNACK</td><td>NET CARBS</td><td>FAT</td><td>CAL</td><td>PROTEIN</td><td></td></tr>
<tr><td></td><td></td><td></td><td></td><td></td><td></td></tr>
<tr><td></td><td></td><td></td><td></td><td></td><td></td></tr>
<tr><td></td><td></td><td></td><td></td><td></td><td></td></tr>
<tr><td></td><td></td><td></td><td></td><td></td><td></td></tr>
<tr><td></td><td></td><td></td><td></td><td></td><td></td></tr>
<tr><td></td><td></td><td></td><td></td><td></td><td></td></tr>
<tr><td></td><td></td><td></td><td></td><td></td><td></td></tr>
<tr><td></td><td></td><td></td><td></td><td></td><td></td></tr>
<tr><td></td><td></td><td></td><td></td><td></td><td></td></tr>
<tr><td></td><td></td><td></td><td></td><td></td><td></td></tr>
<tr><td></td><td></td><td></td><td></td><td></td><td></td></tr>
<tr><td>DAILY GOAL:</td><td></td><td></td><td></td><td></td><td></td></tr>
<tr><td>TOTAL:</td><td></td><td></td><td></td><td></td><td></td></tr>
</table>

MY KETO JOURNEY *Tracker*

SLEEP TRACKER:

DATE _____

 | RISE: | | BEDTIME: | | SLEEP (HRS):

NOTES FOR THE DAY

IN A STATE OF KETOSIS?

YES   NO   UNSURE

WATER INTAKE TRACKER

EXERCISE / WORKOUT ROUTINE

DAILY ENERGY LEVEL

HIGH	**MEDIUM**	**LOW**

BREAKFAST

FAT: CARBS: PROTEIN: CALORIES:

LUNCH

FAT: CARBS: PROTEIN: CALORIES:

DINNER

FAT: CARBS: PROTEIN: CALORIES:

SNACKS

FAT: CARBS: PROTEIN: CALORIES:

TOP 6 PRIORITIES OF THE DAY

END OF THE DAY TOTAL OVERVIEW

CARBS   FAT   PROTEIN   CALORIES

DAILY FOOD *Journal*

FOOD TRACKER

MEAL/SNACK	NET CARBS	FAT	CAL	PROTEIN
DAILY GOAL:				
TOTAL:				

NOTES & MEAL IDEAS

MY KETO JOURNEY *Tracker*

SLEEP TRACKER:

DATE _____

| RISE: | | BEDTIME: | | SLEEP (HRS): |

NOTES FOR THE DAY

_____

_____

_____

IN A STATE OF KETOSIS?

YES   NO   UNSURE

WATER INTAKE TRACKER

EXERCISE / WORKOUT ROUTINE

DAILY ENERGY LEVEL

| **HIGH** | **MEDIUM** | **LOW** |

BREAKFAST

FAT: CARBS: PROTEIN: CALORIES:

LUNCH

FAT: CARBS: PROTEIN: CALORIES:

DINNER

FAT: CARBS: PROTEIN: CALORIES:

SNACKS

FAT: CARBS: PROTEIN: CALORIES:

TOP 6 PRIORITIES OF THE DAY

END OF THE DAY TOTAL OVERVIEW

| CARBS | FAT | PROTEIN | CALORIES |

DAILY FOOD *Journal*

FOOD TRACKER

MEAL/SNACK	NET CARBS	FAT	CAL	PROTEIN
DAILY GOAL:				
TOTAL:				

NOTES & MEAL IDEAS

MY KETO JOURNEY *Tracker*

SLEEP TRACKER:

DATE _____

☼ | RISE: | 🌙 ᶻᶻᶻ | BEDTIME: | 💭ᶻᶻᶻ | SLEEP (HRS):

NOTES FOR THE DAY

_____

_____

_____

EXERCISE / WORKOUT ROUTINE

TOP 6 PRIORITIES OF THE DAY

● _____   ● _____

● _____   ● _____

● _____   ● _____

IN A STATE OF KETOSIS?

YES   NO   UNSURE

WATER INTAKE TRACKER

💧 💧 💧 💧 💧 💧 💧 💧

DAILY ENERGY LEVEL

HIGH   **MEDIUM**   **LOW**

BREAKFAST

FAT: CARBS: PROTEIN: CALORIES:

LUNCH

FAT: CARBS: PROTEIN: CALORIES:

DINNER

FAT: CARBS: PROTEIN: CALORIES:

SNACKS

FAT: CARBS: PROTEIN: CALORIES:

END OF THE DAY TOTAL OVERVIEW

CARBS   FAT   PROTEIN   CALORIES

DAILY FOOD *Journal*

MEAL/SNACK	NET CARBS	FAT	CAL	PROTEIN
DAILY GOAL:				
TOTAL:				

MY KETO JOURNEY *Tracker*

SLEEP TRACKER:

DATE _____

 RISE: | BEDTIME: | SLEEP (HRS):

NOTES FOR THE DAY

_____

_____

_____

EXERCISE / WORKOUT ROUTINE

TOP 6 PRIORITIES OF THE DAY

● _____ ● _____

● _____ ● _____

● _____ ● _____

IN A STATE OF KETOSIS?

YES   NO   UNSURE

WATER INTAKE TRACKER

DAILY ENERGY LEVEL

HIGH	MEDIUM	LOW

BREAKFAST

FAT: CARBS: PROTEIN: CALORIES:

LUNCH

FAT: CARBS: PROTEIN: CALORIES:

DINNER

FAT: CARBS: PROTEIN: CALORIES:

SNACKS

FAT: CARBS: PROTEIN: CALORIES:

END OF THE DAY TOTAL OVERVIEW

CARBS	FAT	PROTEIN	CALORIES

DAILY FOOD *Journal*

FOOD TRACKER

MEAL/SNACK	NET CARBS	FAT	CAL	PROTEIN
DAILY GOAL:				
TOTAL:				

NOTES & MEAL IDEAS

MY KETO JOURNEY *Tracker*

SLEEP TRACKER:

DATE _____

 RISE: | BEDTIME: | SLEEP (HRS):

NOTES FOR THE DAY

_____
_____
_____

EXERCISE / WORKOUT ROUTINE

TOP 6 PRIORITIES OF THE DAY

- ○
- ○
- ○
- ○
- ○
- ○

IN A STATE OF KETOSIS?

YES   NO   UNSURE

WATER INTAKE TRACKER

DAILY ENERGY LEVEL

HIGH	**MEDIUM**	**LOW**

BREAKFAST

FAT: CARBS: PROTEIN: CALORIES:

LUNCH

FAT: CARBS: PROTEIN: CALORIES:

DINNER

FAT: CARBS: PROTEIN: CALORIES:

SNACKS

FAT: CARBS: PROTEIN: CALORIES:

END OF THE DAY TOTAL OVERVIEW

CARBS	FAT	PROTEIN	CALORIES

DAILY FOOD *Journal*

FOOD TRACKER

MEAL/SNACK	NET CARBS	FAT	CAL	PROTEIN
DAILY GOAL:				
TOTAL:				

NOTES & MEAL IDEAS

MY KETO JOURNEY *Tracker*

SLEEP TRACKER:

DATE _____

 RISE: | BEDTIME: | SLEEP (HRS):

NOTES FOR THE DAY

_____

_____

_____

EXERCISE / WORKOUT ROUTINE

TOP 6 PRIORITIES OF THE DAY

● _____ ● _____

● _____ ● _____

● _____ ● _____

IN A STATE OF KETOSIS?

YES   NO   UNSURE

WATER INTAKE TRACKER

DAILY ENERGY LEVEL

HIGH	**MEDIUM**	**LOW**

BREAKFAST

FAT: CARBS: PROTEIN: CALORIES:

LUNCH

FAT: CARBS: PROTEIN: CALORIES:

DINNER

FAT: CARBS: PROTEIN: CALORIES:

SNACKS

FAT: CARBS: PROTEIN: CALORIES:

END OF THE DAY TOTAL OVERVIEW

CARBS	FAT	PROTEIN	CALORIES

DAILY FOOD *Journal*

FOOD TRACKER

MEAL/SNACK	NET CARBS	FAT	CAL	PROTEIN
DAILY GOAL:				
TOTAL:				

NOTES & MEAL IDEAS

MY KETO JOURNEY *Tracker*

SLEEP TRACKER:

DATE _____

☀ | RISE: | 🌙 zᶻᶻ | BEDTIME: | 💭zᶻᶻ | SLEEP (HRS):

NOTES FOR THE DAY

_____
_____
_____

EXERCISE / WORKOUT ROUTINE

TOP 6 PRIORITIES OF THE DAY

• _____ • _____

• _____ • _____

• _____ • _____

IN A STATE OF KETOSIS?

YES   NO   UNSURE

WATER INTAKE TRACKER

💧 💧 💧 💧 💧 💧 💧 💧

DAILY ENERGY LEVEL

HIGH	**MEDIUM**	**LOW**

BREAKFAST

FAT: CARBS: PROTEIN: CALORIES:

LUNCH

FAT: CARBS: PROTEIN: CALORIES:

DINNER

FAT: CARBS: PROTEIN: CALORIES:

SNACKS

FAT: CARBS: PROTEIN: CALORIES:

END OF THE DAY TOTAL OVERVIEW

CARBS	FAT	PROTEIN	CALORIES

DAILY FOOD *Journal*

FOOD TRACKER

MEAL/SNACK	NET CARBS	FAT	CAL	PROTEIN
DAILY GOAL:				
TOTAL:				

NOTES & MEAL IDEAS

MY KETO JOURNEY *Tracker*

SLEEP TRACKER:

DATE _____

| RISE: | | BEDTIME: | | SLEEP (HRS): |

NOTES FOR THE DAY

_____

_____

_____

EXERCISE / WORKOUT ROUTINE

TOP 6 PRIORITIES OF THE DAY

- _____ - _____
- _____ - _____
- _____ - _____

IN A STATE OF KETOSIS?

YES   NO   UNSURE

WATER INTAKE TRACKER

DAILY ENERGY LEVEL

| **HIGH** | **MEDIUM** | **LOW** |

BREAKFAST

FAT: CARBS: PROTEIN: CALORIES:

LUNCH

FAT: CARBS: PROTEIN: CALORIES:

DINNER

FAT: CARBS: PROTEIN: CALORIES:

SNACKS

FAT: CARBS: PROTEIN: CALORIES:

END OF THE DAY TOTAL OVERVIEW

CARBS   FAT   PROTEIN   CALORIES

DAILY FOOD *Journal*

FOOD TRACKER

MEAL/SNACK	NET CARBS	FAT	CAL	PROTEIN
DAILY GOAL:				
TOTAL:				

NOTES & MEAL IDEAS

MY KETO JOURNEY *Tracker*

SLEEP TRACKER:

DATE _____

☀ RISE: _____   🌙 BEDTIME: _____   💭 SLEEP (HRS): _____

NOTES FOR THE DAY

_____
_____
_____

EXERCISE / WORKOUT ROUTINE

TOP 6 PRIORITIES OF THE DAY

- ● _____ ● _____
- ● _____ ● _____
- ● _____ ● _____

IN A STATE OF KETOSIS?

YES   NO   UNSURE

WATER INTAKE TRACKER

💧 💧 💧 💧 💧 💧 💧 💧

DAILY ENERGY LEVEL		
HIGH	**MEDIUM**	**LOW**

BREAKFAST

FAT: CARBS: PROTEIN: CALORIES:

LUNCH

FAT: CARBS: PROTEIN: CALORIES:

DINNER

FAT: CARBS: PROTEIN: CALORIES:

SNACKS

FAT: CARBS: PROTEIN: CALORIES:

END OF THE DAY TOTAL OVERVIEW

CARBS   FAT   PROTEIN   CALORIES

DAILY FOOD *Journal*

FOOD TRACKER

MEAL/SNACK	NET CARBS	FAT	CAL	PROTEIN
DAILY GOAL:				
TOTAL:				

NOTES & MEAL IDEAS

MY KETO JOURNEY *Tracker*

SLEEP TRACKER:

DATE _____

RISE: _____   BEDTIME: _____   SLEEP (HRS): _____

NOTES FOR THE DAY

_____
_____
_____

EXERCISE / WORKOUT ROUTINE

TOP 6 PRIORITIES OF THE DAY

- ○ _____
- ○ _____
- ○ _____

○ _____
○ _____
○ _____

IN A STATE OF KETOSIS?

YES   NO   UNSURE

WATER INTAKE TRACKER

DAILY ENERGY LEVEL

HIGH	**MEDIUM**	**LOW**

BREAKFAST

FAT: CARBS: PROTEIN: CALORIES:

LUNCH

FAT: CARBS: PROTEIN: CALORIES:

DINNER

FAT: CARBS: PROTEIN: CALORIES:

SNACKS

FAT: CARBS: PROTEIN: CALORIES:

END OF THE DAY TOTAL OVERVIEW

CARBS	FAT	PROTEIN	CALORIES

DAILY FOOD *Journal*

FOOD TRACKER

MEAL/SNACK	NET CARBS	FAT	CAL	PROTEIN
DAILY GOAL:				
TOTAL:				

NOTES & MEAL IDEAS

MY KETO JOURNEY *Tracker*

SLEEP TRACKER:

DATE _____

 | RISE: | | BEDTIME: | | SLEEP (HRS): |

NOTES FOR THE DAY

_____

_____

_____

EXERCISE / WORKOUT ROUTINE

TOP 6 PRIORITIES OF THE DAY

- _____   - _____
- _____   - _____
- _____   - _____

IN A STATE OF KETOSIS?

YES   NO   UNSURE

WATER INTAKE TRACKER

DAILY ENERGY LEVEL

HIGH	**MEDIUM**	**LOW**

BREAKFAST

FAT: CARBS: PROTEIN: CALORIES:

LUNCH

FAT: CARBS: PROTEIN: CALORIES:

DINNER

FAT: CARBS: PROTEIN: CALORIES:

SNACKS

FAT: CARBS: PROTEIN: CALORIES:

END OF THE DAY TOTAL OVERVIEW

CARBS	FAT	PROTEIN	CALORIES

DAILY FOOD *Journal*

FOOD TRACKER

MEAL/SNACK	NET CARBS	FAT	CAL	PROTEIN
DAILY GOAL:				
TOTAL:				

NOTES & MEAL IDEAS

MY KETO JOURNEY *Tracker*

SLEEP TRACKER:

DATE _____

 RISE: _____   ☾ᶻᶻᶻ BEDTIME: _____   SLEEP (HRS): _____

NOTES FOR THE DAY

_____

_____

_____

EXERCISE / WORKOUT ROUTINE

TOP 6 PRIORITIES OF THE DAY

● _____   ● _____

● _____   ● _____

● _____   ● _____

IN A STATE OF KETOSIS?

YES   NO   UNSURE

WATER INTAKE TRACKER

💧 💧 💧 💧 💧 💧 💧 💧

DAILY ENERGY LEVEL		
HIGH	**MEDIUM**	**LOW**

BREAKFAST

FAT: CARBS: PROTEIN: CALORIES:

LUNCH

FAT: CARBS: PROTEIN: CALORIES:

DINNER

FAT: CARBS: PROTEIN: CALORIES:

SNACKS

FAT: CARBS: PROTEIN: CALORIES:

END OF THE DAY TOTAL OVERVIEW

CARBS	FAT	PROTEIN	CALORIES

DAILY FOOD *Journal*

FOOD TRACKER

MEAL/SNACK	NET CARBS	FAT	CAL	PROTEIN
DAILY GOAL:				
TOTAL:				

NOTES & MEAL IDEAS

MY KETO JOURNEY *Tracker*

SLEEP TRACKER:

DATE _____

 RISE: _____   ☽ zᵤz BEDTIME: _____   SLEEP (HRS): _____

NOTES FOR THE DAY

_____
_____
_____

EXERCISE / WORKOUT ROUTINE

TOP 6 PRIORITIES OF THE DAY

- ● _____   ● _____
- ● _____   ● _____
- ● _____   ● _____

IN A STATE OF KETOSIS?

YES   NO   UNSURE

WATER INTAKE TRACKER

💧 💧 💧 💧 💧 💧 💧

DAILY ENERGY LEVEL

HIGH	MEDIUM	LOW

BREAKFAST

FAT: CARBS: PROTEIN: CALORIES:

LUNCH

FAT: CARBS: PROTEIN: CALORIES:

DINNER

FAT: CARBS: PROTEIN: CALORIES:

SNACKS

FAT: CARBS: PROTEIN: CALORIES:

END OF THE DAY TOTAL OVERVIEW

CARBS	FAT	PROTEIN	CALORIES

DAILY FOOD *Journal*

MEAL/SNACK	NET CARBS	FAT	CAL	PROTEIN
DAILY GOAL:				
TOTAL:				

MY KETO JOURNEY *Tracker*

SLEEP TRACKER:

 RISE:

DATE _____

🌙 BEDTIME:

 SLEEP (HRS):

NOTES FOR THE DAY

....
....
....

EXERCISE / WORKOUT ROUTINE

IN A STATE OF KETOSIS?

YES   NO   UNSURE

WATER INTAKE TRACKER

DAILY ENERGY LEVEL

HIGH	MEDIUM	LOW

BREAKFAST

FAT: CARBS: PROTEIN: CALORIES:

LUNCH

FAT: CARBS: PROTEIN: CALORIES:

DINNER

FAT: CARBS: PROTEIN: CALORIES:

SNACKS

FAT: CARBS: PROTEIN: CALORIES:

TOP 6 PRIORITIES OF THE DAY

END OF THE DAY TOTAL OVERVIEW

CARBS	FAT	PROTEIN	CALORIES

DAILY FOOD *Journal*

MEAL/SNACK	NET CARBS	FAT	CAL	PROTEIN
DAILY GOAL:				
TOTAL:				

NOTES & MEAL IDEAS

MY KETO JOURNEY *Tracker*

SLEEP TRACKER:

DATE _____

☀ | RISE: | 🌙 zzz | BEDTIME: | ☁zzz | SLEEP (HRS):

NOTES FOR THE DAY

_____

_____

_____

EXERCISE / WORKOUT ROUTINE

TOP 6 PRIORITIES OF THE DAY

● _____ ● _____

● _____ ● _____

● _____ ● _____

IN A STATE OF KETOSIS?

YES   NO   UNSURE

WATER INTAKE TRACKER

💧 💧 💧 💧 💧 💧 💧 💧

DAILY ENERGY LEVEL

HIGH	**MEDIUM**	**LOW**

BREAKFAST

FAT: CARBS: PROTEIN: CALORIES:

LUNCH

FAT: CARBS: PROTEIN: CALORIES:

DINNER

FAT: CARBS: PROTEIN: CALORIES:

SNACKS

FAT: CARBS: PROTEIN: CALORIES:

END OF THE DAY TOTAL OVERVIEW

CARBS	FAT	PROTEIN	CALORIES

DAILY FOOD *Journal*

FOOD TRACKER

MEAL/SNACK	NET CARBS	FAT	CAL	PROTEIN
DAILY GOAL:				
TOTAL:				

NOTES & MEAL IDEAS

MY KETO JOURNEY *Tracker*

SLEEP TRACKER:

DATE _____

| RISE: | | BEDTIME: | | SLEEP (HRS): |

NOTES FOR THE DAY

_____

_____

_____

EXERCISE / WORKOUT ROUTINE

TOP 6 PRIORITIES OF THE DAY

- ● _____ ● _____
- ● _____ ● _____
- ● _____ ● _____

IN A STATE OF KETOSIS?

YES   NO   UNSURE

WATER INTAKE TRACKER

DAILY ENERGY LEVEL

| **HIGH** | **MEDIUM** | **LOW** |

BREAKFAST

FAT: CARBS: PROTEIN: CALORIES:

LUNCH

FAT: CARBS: PROTEIN: CALORIES:

DINNER

FAT: CARBS: PROTEIN: CALORIES:

SNACKS

FAT: CARBS: PROTEIN: CALORIES:

END OF THE DAY TOTAL OVERVIEW

CARBS	FAT	PROTEIN	CALORIES

DAILY FOOD *Journal*

FOOD TRACKER

MEAL/SNACK	NET CARBS	FAT	CAL	PROTEIN
DAILY GOAL:				
TOTAL:				

NOTES & MEAL IDEAS

90-DAY

You Did It!

Progress

Weight and Measurements

Chest

Arm

Waist

Hips

Thigh

FINAL MEASUREMENTS:

WEIGHT:

LEFT ARM:

RIGHT ARM:

CHEST:

WAIST:

HIPS:

LEFT THIGH:

RIGHT THIGH:

My Journey

THOUGHTS ON MY KETO JOURNEY:

My KETO Recipes

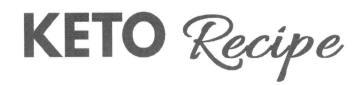

RECIPE NAME:

	Keto	Low Carb	Paleo	Vegetarian	Vegan	Dairy Free	Gluten Free
	☐	☐	☐	☐	☐	☐	☐

QTY	INGREDIENTS

RECIPE INSTRUCTIONS

NOTES & RECIPE REVIEW

Serves	
Prep Time	
Cook Time	
Tools	
Temp	

	Carbs	Fat	Protein	Cals
Total				

KETO *Recipe*

RECIPE NAME:

	Keto	Low Carb	Paleo	Vegetarian	Vegan	Dairy Free	Gluten Free
	☐	☐	☐	☐	☐	☐	☐

QTY	INGREDIENTS	RECIPE INSTRUCTIONS

NOTES & RECIPE REVIEW

Serves	
Prep Time	
Cook Time	
Tools	
Temp	

	Carbs	Fat	Protein	Cals
Total				

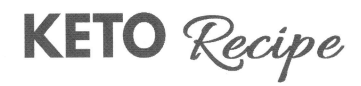

KETO *Recipe*

RECIPE NAME:

	Keto	Low Carb	Paleo	Vegetarian	Vegan	Dairy Free	Gluten Free
	☐	☐	☐	☐	☐	☐	☐

QTY	INGREDIENTS	RECIPE INSTRUCTIONS

NOTES & RECIPE REVIEW

Serves	
Prep Time	
Cook Time	
Tools	
Temp	

	Carbs	Fat	Protein	Cals
Total				

KETO *Recipe*

RECIPE NAME:

Keto	Low Carb	Paleo	Vegetarian	Vegan	Dairy Free	Gluten Free
☐	☐	☐	☐	☐	☐	☐

QTY	INGREDIENTS	RECIPE INSTRUCTIONS

NOTES & RECIPE REVIEW

Serves	
Prep Time	
Cook Time	
Tools	
Temp	

	Carbs	Fat	Protein	Cals
Total				

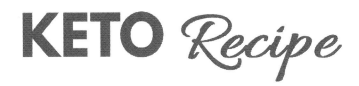

KETO *Recipe*

RECIPE NAME:

Keto	Low Carb	Paleo	Vegetarian	Vegan	Dairy Free	Gluten Free
☐	☐	☐	☐	☐	☐	☐

QTY	INGREDIENTS	RECIPE INSTRUCTIONS

NOTES & RECIPE REVIEW

Serves	
Prep Time	
Cook Time	
Tools	
Temp	

	Carbs	Fat	Protein	Cals
Total				

KETO *Recipe*

RECIPE NAME:

	Keto	Low Carb	Paleo	Vegetarian	Vegan	Dairy Free	Gluten Free
	☐	☐	☐	☐	☐	☐	☐

QTY	INGREDIENTS	RECIPE INSTRUCTIONS

NOTES & RECIPE REVIEW

Serves	
Prep Time	
Cook Time	
Tools	
Temp	

	Carbs	Fat	Protein	Cals
Total				

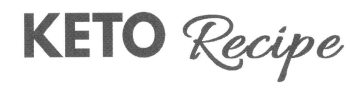

RECIPE NAME:

Keto	Low Carb	Paleo	Vegetarian	Vegan	Dairy Free	Gluten Free
☐	☐	☐	☐	☐	☐	☐

QTY	INGREDIENTS

RECIPE INSTRUCTIONS

NOTES & RECIPE REVIEW

Serves	
Prep Time	
Cook Time	
Tools	
Temp	

	Carbs	Fat	Protein	Cals
Total				

KETO *Recipe*

RECIPE NAME:

	Keto	Low Carb	Paleo	Vegetarian	Vegan	Dairy Free	Gluten Free
	☐	☐	☐	☐	☐	☐	☐

QTY	INGREDIENTS

RECIPE INSTRUCTIONS

NOTES & RECIPE REVIEW

Serves	
Prep Time	
Cook Time	
Tools	
Temp	

	Carbs	Fat	Protein	Cals
Total				

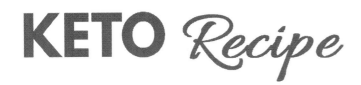

KETO *Recipe*

RECIPE NAME:
_____

	Keto	Low Carb	Paleo	Vegetarian	Vegan	Dairy Free	Gluten Free
	☐	☐	☐	☐	☐	☐	☐

QTY	INGREDIENTS

RECIPE INSTRUCTIONS

NOTES & RECIPE REVIEW

Serves	
Prep Time	
Cook Time	
Tools	
Temp	

	Carbs	Fat	Protein	Cals
Total				

KETO *Recipe*

RECIPE NAME:

	Keto	Low Carb	Paleo	Vegetarian	Vegan	Dairy Free	Gluten Free
	☐	☐	☐	☐	☐	☐	☐

QTY	INGREDIENTS	RECIPE INSTRUCTIONS

NOTES & RECIPE REVIEW	
	Serves
	Prep Time
	Cook Time
	Tools
	Temp

	Carbs	Fat	Protein	Cals
Total				

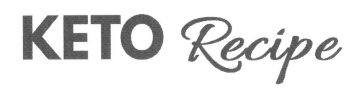

KETO *Recipe*

RECIPE NAME:

	Keto	Low Carb	Paleo	Vegetarian	Vegan	Dairy Free	Gluten Free
	☐	☐	☐	☐	☐	☐	☐

QTY	INGREDIENTS	RECIPE INSTRUCTIONS

NOTES & RECIPE REVIEW		
	Serves	
	Prep Time	
	Cook Time	
	Tools	
	Temp	

	Carbs	Fat	Protein	Cals
Total				

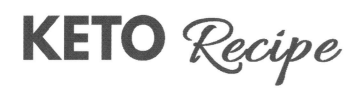

KETO *Recipe*

RECIPE NAME:

Keto	Low Carb	Paleo	Vegetarian	Vegan	Dairy Free	Gluten Free
☐	☐	☐	☐	☐	☐	☐

QTY	INGREDIENTS	RECIPE INSTRUCTIONS

NOTES & RECIPE REVIEW

Serves	
Prep Time	
Cook Time	
Tools	
Temp	

	Carbs	Fat	Protein	Cals
Total				

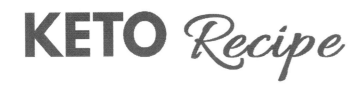

KETO *Recipe*

RECIPE NAME:

	Keto	Low Carb	Paleo	Vegetarian	Vegan	Dairy Free	Gluten Free
	☐	☐	☐	☐	☐	☐	☐

QTY	INGREDIENTS

RECIPE INSTRUCTIONS

NOTES & RECIPE REVIEW

Serves	
Prep Time	
Cook Time	
Tools	
Temp	

	Carbs	Fat	Protein	Cals
Total				

KETO *Recipe*

RECIPE NAME:

	Keto	Low Carb	Paleo	Vegetarian	Vegan	Dairy Free	Gluten Free
	☐	☐	☐	☐	☐	☐	☐

QTY	INGREDIENTS	RECIPE INSTRUCTIONS

NOTES & RECIPE REVIEW		

Serves	
Prep Time	
Cook Time	
Tools	
Temp	

	Carbs	Fat	Protein	Cals
Total				

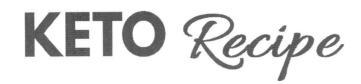

KETO *Recipe*

RECIPE NAME:
_____

Keto	Low Carb	Paleo	Vegetarian	Vegan	Dairy Free	Gluten Free
☐	☐	☐	☐	☐	☐	☐

QTY	INGREDIENTS

RECIPE INSTRUCTIONS

NOTES & RECIPE REVIEW

Serves	
Prep Time	
Cook Time	
Tools	
Temp	

	Carbs	Fat	Protein	Cals
Total				

KETO *Recipe*

RECIPE NAME:

Keto	Low Carb	Paleo	Vegetarian	Vegan	Dairy Free	Gluten Free
☐	☐	☐	☐	☐	☐	☐

QTY	INGREDIENTS

RECIPE INSTRUCTIONS

NOTES & RECIPE REVIEW

Serves	
Prep Time	
Cook Time	
Tools	
Temp	

	Carbs	Fat	Protein	Cals
Total				

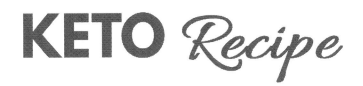

KETO *Recipe*

RECIPE NAME:

	Keto	Low Carb	Paleo	Vegetarian	Vegan	Dairy Free	Gluten Free
	☐	☐	☐	☐	☐	☐	☐

QTY	INGREDIENTS	RECIPE INSTRUCTIONS

NOTES & RECIPE REVIEW

Serves	
Prep Time	
Cook Time	
Tools	
Temp	

	Carbs	Fat	Protein	Cals
Total				

KETO *Recipe*

RECIPE NAME:

	Keto	Low Carb	Paleo	Vegetarian	Vegan	Dairy Free	Gluten Free
	☐	☐	☐	☐	☐	☐	☐

QTY	INGREDIENTS

RECIPE INSTRUCTIONS

NOTES & RECIPE REVIEW

Serves	
Prep Time	
Cook Time	
Tools	
Temp	

	Carbs	Fat	Protein	Cals
Total				

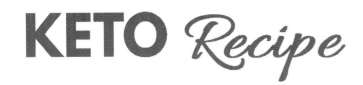

KETO Recipe

RECIPE NAME:

Keto	Low Carb	Paleo	Vegetarian	Vegan	Dairy Free	Gluten Free
☐	☐	☐	☐	☐	☐	☐

QTY	INGREDIENTS

RECIPE INSTRUCTIONS

NOTES & RECIPE REVIEW

Serves	
Prep Time	
Cook Time	
Tools	
Temp	

	Carbs	Fat	Protein	Cals
Total				

KETO *Recipe*

RECIPE NAME:

Keto	Low Carb	Paleo	Vegetarian	Vegan	Dairy Free	Gluten Free
☐	☐	☐	☐	☐	☐	☐

QTY	INGREDIENTS	RECIPE INSTRUCTIONS

NOTES & RECIPE REVIEW

Serves	
Prep Time	
Cook Time	
Tools	
Temp	

	Carbs	Fat	Protein	Cals
Total				

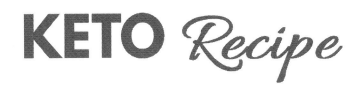
KETO *Recipe*

RECIPE NAME:

Keto	Low Carb	Paleo	Vegetarian	Vegan	Dairy Free	Gluten Free
☐	☐	☐	☐	☐	☐	☐

QTY	INGREDIENTS

RECIPE INSTRUCTIONS

NOTES & RECIPE REVIEW

Serves	
Prep Time	
Cook Time	
Tools	
Temp	

	Carbs	Fat	Protein	Cals
Total				

KETO *Recipe*

RECIPE NAME:

	Keto	Low Carb	Paleo	Vegetarian	Vegan	Dairy Free	Gluten Free
	☐	☐	☐	☐	☐	☐	☐

QTY	INGREDIENTS	RECIPE INSTRUCTIONS

NOTES & RECIPE REVIEW

Serves	
Prep Time	
Cook Time	
Tools	
Temp	

	Carbs	Fat	Protein	Cals
Total				

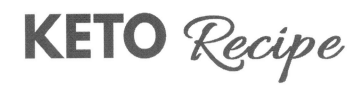

KETO Recipe

RECIPE NAME:

Keto	Low Carb	Paleo	Vegetarian	Vegan	Dairy Free	Gluten Free
☐	☐	☐	☐	☐	☐	☐

QTY	INGREDIENTS

RECIPE INSTRUCTIONS

NOTES & RECIPE REVIEW

Serves	
Prep Time	
Cook Time	
Tools	
Temp	

	Carbs	Fat	Protein	Cals
Total				

KETO *Recipe*

RECIPE NAME:

	Keto	Low Carb	Paleo	Vegetarian	Vegan	Dairy Free	Gluten Free
	☐	☐	☐	☐	☐	☐	☐

QTY	INGREDIENTS	RECIPE INSTRUCTIONS

NOTES & RECIPE REVIEW		
	Serves	
	Prep Time	
	Cook Time	
	Tools	
	Temp	

	Carbs	Fat	Protein	Cals
Total				

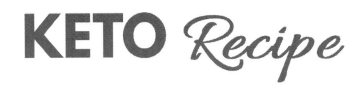

KETO *Recipe*

RECIPE NAME:

	Keto	Low Carb	Paleo	Vegetarian	Vegan	Dairy Free	Gluten Free
	☐	☐	☐	☐	☐	☐	☐

QTY	INGREDIENTS	RECIPE INSTRUCTIONS

NOTES & RECIPE REVIEW		

Serves	
Prep Time	
Cook Time	
Tools	
Temp	

	Carbs	Fat	Protein	Cals
Total				

KETO *Recipe*

RECIPE NAME:
_____

	Keto	Low Carb	Paleo	Vegetarian	Vegan	Dairy Free	Gluten Free
	☐	☐	☐	☐	☐	☐	☐

QTY	INGREDIENTS

RECIPE INSTRUCTIONS

NOTES & RECIPE REVIEW

Serves	
Prep Time	
Cook Time	
Tools	
Temp	

	Carbs	Fat	Protein	Cals
Total				

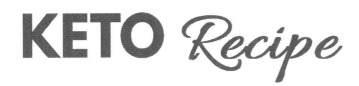

KETO *Recipe*

RECIPE NAME:

Keto	Low Carb	Paleo	Vegetarian	Vegan	Dairy Free	Gluten Free
☐	☐	☐	☐	☐	☐	☐

QTY	INGREDIENTS

RECIPE INSTRUCTIONS

NOTES & RECIPE REVIEW

Serves	
Prep Time	
Cook Time	
Tools	
Temp	

	Carbs	Fat	Protein	Cals
Total				

KETO *Recipe*

RECIPE NAME:

	Keto	Low Carb	Paleo	Vegetarian	Vegan	Dairy Free	Gluten Free
	☐	☐	☐	☐	☐	☐	☐

QTY	INGREDIENTS

RECIPE INSTRUCTIONS

NOTES & RECIPE REVIEW

Serves	
Prep Time	
Cook Time	
Tools	
Temp	

	Carbs	Fat	Protein	Cals
Total				

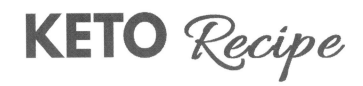

RECIPE NAME:

	Keto	Low Carb	Paleo	Vegetarian	Vegan	Dairy Free	Gluten Free
	☐	☐	☐	☐	☐	☐	☐

QTY	INGREDIENTS	RECIPE INSTRUCTIONS

NOTES & RECIPE REVIEW		Serves	
		Prep Time	
		Cook Time	
		Tools	
		Temp	

	Carbs	Fat	Protein	Cals
Total				

KETO *Recipe*

RECIPE NAME:
_____

Keto	Low Carb	Paleo	Vegetarian	Vegan	Dairy Free	Gluten Free
☐	☐	☐	☐	☐	☐	☐

QTY	INGREDIENTS	RECIPE INSTRUCTIONS

NOTES & RECIPE REVIEW		
	Serves	
	Prep Time	
	Cook Time	
	Tools	
	Temp	

	Carbs	Fat	Protein	Cals
Total				

Made in the USA
Monee, IL
05 September 2022

13291676R00127